Wondey Made

The Dr. Francis Joel Smith, PhD Story

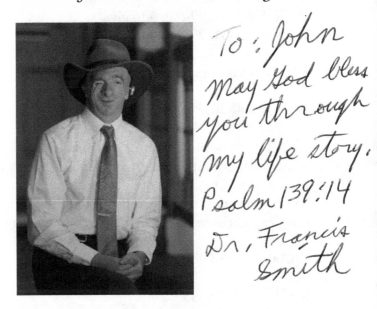

Image by: Kenn Bisio, 2018

Treacher Collins syndrome—
the amazing, extremely unique life journey of
Dr. Francis Joel Smith, PhD
from 1975 to 2012

Michele DuBroy and Francis Smith

ISBN 978-1-64299-804-7 (paperback)
ISBN 978-1-64299-805-4 (digital)
ISBN 978-1-64299-858-0 (hardcover)

Library of Congress Control Number: 2018948326

Christian Faith Publishing, Inc.
832 Park Avenue
Meadville, PA 16335
www.christianfaithpublishing.com

This is a work of non-fiction. At the discretion of the publisher, some names have been changed to protect privacy. Personal information from interviews, written documents, phone conversations, and e-mails regarding Dr. Smith have been added, along with adaptations of certain memories to enhance the story.

All photos used in this publication are from Dr. Francis Smith's personal collection or were taken by Michele DuBroy and are courtesy of Dr. Smith or family members and Michele DuBroy exclusively for this publication. Kenn Bisio did all cover photos.

Printed in the United States of America

Betty Johnson Smith

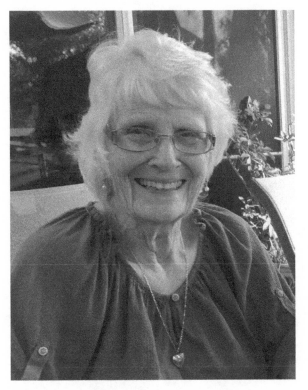

Image by Michele DuBroy, 2016

This book is dedicated to my mother, Betty Johnson Smith, who opened her heart and home to me and ten other children, all of us with unique challenges, and raised us all in the love of the LORD. I remain close to her to this day.

—Dr. Francis Joel Smith, PhD

I will praise thee;
for I am fearfully and wonderfully made:
marvelous are thy works
and that my soul knoweth right well.

—Psalm 139:14

Contents

Book 1

Ephesians 1:11–12 and Matthew 6:31–33

Chapter 1

God Is in All Things

Chapter 2

God's Sovereignty in Motion

Chapter 3

Song of Solomon

Book 2

Jeremiah 29:11

Book 3

Psalm 63:8

Chapter 4
Let the Healing Begin

Book 4
1 Thessalonians 4:13

Chapter 1
An Unexpected Farewell

Chapter 2

Chapter 3

Unwavering Faith

Chapter 4

The Longest Yard

Book 5

Proverbs 3:5–6

Chapter 1

Ireland—Home Sweet Ancestral Home

Chapter 2

The LORD Reveals His Will

Book 6
Joshua 1:9

Chapter 1
The Journey of a Lifetime

Chapter 2

Book 7
Psalm 139

Foreword

The sacredness of life is basic to all of creation. Human life is the crowning manifestation of that sacredness.

You are about to read an amazing account concerning a life that, under today's cultural values, would have been discarded at its beginning without hesitation. It is the life of Francis Joel Smith.

The treasure of this man's life is very evident to all who know him. But his capacity for life, his love for God, his selfless relationships with his peers, and his most unusual gifts and abilities did not become evident except through a long difficult series of unbelievable personal experiences in his life.

At the beginning, there was absolutely no hope. Through his early years, there was only suffering, pain, and an endless need for help beyond medical capabilities. Many would question why God would allow anyone to endure such difficulties.

In the providence of a great and loving God, His love and care were found in the hearts of several key players. These special angels of ministry loved Francis and cared for him as a precious life valued by God. And they recognized this value. With great personal sacrifice and painstaking care, they ministered to him in his early years and through the years to follow.

In my many years as a pastor, I have never met or known anyone more vibrant, delightful, or persevering than Francis. His love for God and his desire to make a significant contribution to those who share in his kind of suffering is an example without equal.

You will be blessed, challenged, and humbled as you go with him on a most unusual journey through his lifetime from its very beginning. The imprints of the hand of God are all over his life. His future is bright and promises to be fruitful and a blessing to all whose lives he will touch.

And you will also be greatly encouraged! Read on!

—Dr. Pastor David C. Innes
Hamilton Square Baptist Church
San Francisco, California

Treacher Collins Syndrome

Treacher Collins syndrome (mandibulofacial dysostosis and Franceschetti-Zwalen-Klein syndrome) is a rare genetic condition affecting the way the face—especially the jaw, cheekbones, ears, and eyelids—develops during the first trimester of pregnancy. These differences often cause problems with breathing, swallowing, chewing, hearing, and speech.

Prologue

San Francisco, California
August 2012

Francis Joel Smith, thirty-seven, stood in front of his bathroom mirror, looking carefully at a face that belied his nerves. Reflecting was a miraculous face that had endured over twenty surgeries in just as many years in order to give him some semblance of as normal of a face, and life, as possible.

In a few hours, Francis was going to give his oral dissertation for his doctorate in oral and craniofacial sciences in front of his professors and peers at the University of California San Francisco (UCSF) campus, and his stomach was filled with butterflies. In the audience would be Dr. Ralph Marcucio, his supervising professor; Dr. John Greenspan, his academic and personal adviser; and Drs. Dan Ramos and Rich Schneider. Also among them would be his future boss and mentor, Dr. Benedikt Hallgrimsson, from the University of Calgary, Canada, who was on his dissertation committee. There were even a few special friends who were members from his church, expected. Sadly, the two most important people in his life, his mother

Betty Smith and his younger sister Ruth, were unable to travel from Fort Wayne, Indiana, to be there with him. To keep them close to him for this occasion, Francis wore his favorite shirt from Ireland his mother had given to him. After fourteen years in college, and the last five of them at UCSF, he was to achieve his years-long dream of becoming a doctor of philosophy (PhD) in craniofacial research. For years, he had dreamed about being able to help others who were afflicted with a craniofacial disorder as he was. This was a wonderful day!

On the bed stand next to Francis's bed was his Bible. Thanks to his adoptive parents, Bob and Betty Smith, who had raised him and his siblings on the Word, God's promises had been instilled in him from the time he was two and a half years old. The Bible's words of truth and wisdom faithfully carried him through the good times and the bad.

Francis sat down for a moment and opened the book. His one good eye focused on one of his favorite verses, Jeremiah 29:11: "'For I know the plans I have for you,' declares the LORD, 'plans to prosper you and not to harm you, plans to give you hope and a future.'"

Francis pondered the verse for a moment. A sense of calm came over him, and for the next few moments, he reflected on his life. Oh, how far the LORD had carried him, he thought to himself. Born with Treacher Collins syndrome (TCS), a rare genetic disorder that affects the forming of the craniofacial structures during the first trimester of pregnancy, he was documented as one of the worst known cases in the medical world at that time. Its origins were in the United Kingdom and afflicted very light-skinned people, and very little was known about this disorder in the United States. He was so badly malformed at birth no one expected him to live, but the LORD had His own extraordinary plans in place for him from the moment he was conceived; thus, countless others would see God's miraculous work in Francis's life. Physically frail and deemed "retarded" because he initially couldn't hear or speak, he was later on proven to possess a genius IQ and an outgoing, loving personality.

Francis leaned back in his chair and stared blankly at the ceiling. He had a strong desire to examine his heart. Aside from the love he felt for his family and his Savior Jesus Christ, the questions foremost in his mind were as follows: Was the LORD glorified by his life? Had he loved his neighbor as Christ loved him? What about forgiving those who wronged him? Had he truly forgiven them as Christ had forgiven him? Was Jesus always first in his life, ahead of anything or anyone else? When it came to the LORD's perfect will for his life, had he willingly submitted, or did he continually battle for his own desires? Had he sought the lost and led them to Christ? Could he claim obedience to His Word? Did others see Jesus in him? Was he thankful for how the LORD had knitted him in his mother's womb instead of seeing his challenges as a curse? Had how he handled his challenges blessed others? The list was endless.

Francis briefly dozed off. The memories…

We know that for those who
Love God all things
Work together for good

—Romans 8:28

Preface

God had a very special plan for my life. I am uniquely, fearfully, and wonderfully made by the hands of the Master Artist Himself (Psalm 139:14). I was not expected to live when born, much less speak, hear, or lead a normal life; but with the help of God, my forever family, doctors, and friends, I have fought hard and persevered to overcome my trials. My foster mother in Indianapolis, Mrs. Collins, was an "angel unaware" that God used to save my life while she cared for me for my first two and a half years of life. My adoptive parents, Bob and Betty Smith, who also adopted ten other children with special needs over the course of their marriage, gave us the tools to live good lives to serve others. But more importantly, my parents taught us to trust God's Son Jesus Christ for salvation and serve Him in our lives. My pastors and church families have reinforced my growing faith over my lifetime. My trials (surgeries, medical issues, facing social attitudes and bullying, among others) were used by God to strengthen my faith, teach me to persevere, and instill compassion for others facing similar challenges later in my life. I also have had to wait patiently, trusting the sovereign will of God to lead me to the next steps of my life's journey. He has also used the encouragement of my family, friends, and mentors to guide me along my path and shape my distinct career of craniofacial research and outreach. In short, my unique life experience with craniofacial anomalies has been divinely used to give me the heart to encourage others facing craniofacial anomalies and other challenges. It is my hope that my life story will inspire others to never give up on overcoming their challenges and trust God's leading in their lives.

—Francis

Acknowledgments

No one writes a publication of this magnitude alone. When it became known that Francis intended to publish his story, so many wonderful people who were a part of his (especially) earlier years came forward to share their personal memories.

With very special thanks to Betty Smith, Ruth Smith, Lee Durland, Sarah Litch, Myra Kidd, and Keith Wittebols for sharing their memories and contributions. And for Francis's siblings, Rob and James, who also allowed their names and stories to be used although they were not interviewed.

We would also like to thank Dr. Pastor David C. Innes of Hamilton Square Baptist Church in San Francisco for being our caring and giving pastor. To Drs. Ralph Marcucio, John Greenspan, and Daniel Ramos from University of California San Francisco for taking Francis into their educational and research fold and for caring so much about him. And in Canada, to Dr. Benedikt Hallgrimsson, who was always a supporter and admirer and gave Francis his first postdoctorate research job.

My friends were supportive as well. With special thanks to Ingrid Hart who shares my passion for getting

23

the "write" job done and for her ongoing suggestions and guidance when I couldn't see the forest through the trees. To Christa and Steve Vetter who encouraged me to keep moving forward after several setbacks; for our fellowship group at the home of Don and Georgetta Quiring who collectively kept us in prayer, and for Lydia Normand Rhine who put up with my long disappearances when I went "down under" for days and sometimes weeks at a time. And to Deborah Innes Kelly, a pastor's daughter and a pastor's wife, and fellow writer. Deborah, you are a true example of a godly woman with a true and tireless servants heart, and I am blessed to know you. Thank you for your wisdom through some difficult trials. You are loved. For my Aunt, Carol Clayton Harris; I could not have made it through the last few years without you. I am so grateful for your love, generosity, and presence in my life. To my cousins, Moses and Colleen Avila and their children who constantly kept this story in prayer. Not to mention our church family at Hamilton Square, so many of whom rarely failed to ask how the book was coming along. I would especially like to acknowledge Vickie Hocking and her mother Barbara Pittman, two of my longest tried and true friends. Vickie has suffered from polio from the time she was barely a toddler, and her grace and perseverance displayed in a challenged and difficult life is an inspiration to all who know her.

For Cher, who selflessly lends her love, dedication, and celebrity, along with her passion for outreach that she and Francis share with the wonderful and outstanding craniofacial community.

And especially for my mom, Margaret, who raised me to love God. She is home with the LORD.

Book 1

*In him we are also chosen, having been predestined
according to the plan of him who works out
everything in conformity with the purpose of his will,
in order that we, who were the first to put our hope
in Christ, might be for the praise of his glory.*

—Ephesians 1:11–12

*Therefore, do not be anxious, saying,
"What shall we eat?" or "What shall we wear?"
For the Gentiles seek after all these things,
and your heavenly Father
knows that you need them all.
But seek first the kingdom of God
and his righteousness,
and all these things will be added to you.*

—Matthew 6:31–33

Chapter 1

God Is in All Things
1975–1977

God's Amazing Hand

April 25, 1975, was a gorgeous spring day in the university town of Bloomington, Indiana. At fifty-eight degrees, it was still a bit on the chilly side, but after the long harsh winter, the majestic palette of vibrant spring colors gently unfolding across the heartland marked a welcomed rejuvenation of body, mind, and spirit.

Everywhere you looked, the outdoors was alive with people walking, biking, and standing on the sidewalk, talking. What mattered was that they were outdoors, breathing in the fresh springtime air. The sky was blue; the clouds were white and puffy. The birds were singing, and the bees were pollinating. It was a perfect day.

Mr. and Mrs. O'Connor, who were both professors from a university in Ireland, had come to the Indianapolis, Indiana, area for their one-year sabbatical. Much to their surprise, they conceived during this time, and now they were juggling to get back home in time for their child, their first, to be born. Early that morning and quite unexpectedly, Mrs. O'Connor went into premature labor. A short while later, she was admitted to Bloomington Hospital. While her nervous husband paced in the waiting room, she was wheeled into the delivery room. There is always concern when a labor is premature, and the obstetrics and gynecology (OB-GYN) staff was well prepared for the unexpected. However, what happened next horrified everyone. As the newborn began to emerge from the birth canal, the doctor turned its head to guide it out of its mother. Only then was he able to see that the infant's tiny face was severely malformed. Where there should have been prominent, well-formed outer ears and ear canals, there were only tiny skin tags and no ear canal openings at all. The more the infant emerged from its mother's body, the worse it got. The infant's face lacked any semblance of a chin, and as a result, its lower jaw was so tiny that its mouth hung wide open, and its large tongue protruded from its mouth. Inside its mouth, there was no palate, just a huge gaping cleft palate. Its face was sunken due to the lack of the arch-shaped skull bones that form the cheeks, and the eyes had no eye sockets for support. Instead, they were sunken and rolled around in their holes in its tiny undersized skull. A nurse gasped; another let out a small cry.

The rest of its body emerged quickly. It was a boy. His tiny body was so emaciated the overhead surgical light shone straight through him. Within moments, he began to have severe difficulty breathing, caused by a tongue that was too big for his mouth and fell back into his throat obstructing the airway. Both his mouth and throat were abnormally small. The birth of this innocent, horribly deformed infant boy was a shock for all concerned.

The mother moaned and twisted in response to the sudden chaos before she started frantically yelling for her baby. The delivery team jumped into action, simultaneously to keep the baby alive and to calm the frightened, hysterical mother. Although emergency procedures saved his life, there was very little hope the baby would survive.

Once the O'Connors were reunited in her hospital room, without their baby, the devastated couple was faced with an agonizing decision. Their newborn son could not survive the trip back to Ireland. The severe abnormalities of his facial structure and other life-threatening complications made it next to impossible for him to be taken anywhere other than to a specialized hospital where he would receive around-the-clock care. His expectancy to live was practically nonexistent.

Time was now critical. Newborn O'Connor needed urgent medical care beyond what could be done on an emergency basis at the birth hospital. With tremendous sorrow, the O'Connors were faced with a devastating choice. They could remain together as a family until he died, trusting he would be kept as comfortable as possible. Beyond that, they knew they could not possibly care for him. Surely, his medical care would be in the hundreds of thousands of dollars, or possibly even more, over time. Adding to the complication was the fact they were not even United States citizens. Their son's best chance for survival would be for him to become a ward of the state of Indiana. The state would see to it he got the best medical care medically possible, and if he survived and gained strength, he would even be eligible for adoption.

Heartbroken and guilt ridden, the O'Connors relinquished all parental rights. As their final act as his parents, they named their firstborn son, Hugh Dermott O'Connor, the name on his birth certificate. From that point on, nothing more is known about infant Hugh's birth parents. One can only imagine the grief and the guilt they must have felt as they went forward with their lives without their firstborn son.

Thus began the miraculous unfolding of God's predestined plan for a newborn whose life would touch so many other lives in a way that gave God the Father all the glory.

A Disheartening Diagnosis

As quickly as the necessary documents were in place, Hugh was transferred to James Whitcomb Riley Hospital for Children in Indianapolis, Indiana, where the fight for his life began in earnest. This highly renowned children's hospital is dedicated to the care of children who suffer from all kinds of acute and rare illnesses. Immediately upon arrival, he was placed in a special intensive care unit designed for newborns with severe and life-threatening medical problems such as birth defects, inherited diseases, and other serious illnesses. Their dedication to this parentless new-born fighting so valiantly for his life was as immediate as it was extraordinary. No sooner had the beleaguered new-born settled in than almost immediately, he experienced several near-fatal episodes of obstructive respiratory arrest. Less than twenty-four hours old, Hugh was rushed into the operating room where doctors had to surgically create a tracheostomy, an opening in his throat where a special custom-made 000-size sterling silver tracheostomy tube or "trach" was inserted to help him breathe. The smallest manufactured size available was a 00, and even that was too large. There were no parents who loved him weeping over his incubator. Instead, those who lovingly helped him hold on and fight for his life were a team of dedicated professionals who were doing everything possible so this little guy could live. There wasn't one among them who worked so fervently to save him who hadn't fallen in love with him.

Once Hugh's breathing was stabilized, teams of doctors and medical geneticists began the grueling rituals of testing in order to accurately diagnose all of this infant's multiple and life-threatening medical problems.

Hugh was diagnosed with Treacher Collins syndrome (TCS), a rare genetic craniofacial disorder that was also known as mandibulofacial dysostosis. This very rare syndrome occurs mostly among light-skinned children and is so rare many American doctors had, at that time, never heard of it, let alone encountered anyone affected by it. It has its origins in lighter-skinned people who fare from the British Isles. Initially, this disorder was believed to be purely genetic, but as craniofacial abnormalities appeared to be on the rise in infants whose parents do not possess this gene, it is now widely believed the syndrome is often the result of spontaneous mutation in the first, and most critical, first trimester of pregnancy. Baby Hugh's parents were Irish, so it is believed that his is genetic, meaning that if he someday chooses to conceive naturally, there is a 50 percent chance he will pass this gene onto his own children. On all fronts, this was not good news.

For the next few months, Riley Hospital was Infant O'Connor's home while his medical team struggled with what they could do medically for him not only immediately but for his future as well. What amazed them all was how this tiny, emaciated, deformed infant struggled and fought to stay alive. All were in agreement; there was something special about him, very, very special. There wasn't a nurse, an aide, or a doctor who cared for him who hadn't fallen in love with him.

Their immediate concern was to get the proper nourishment into him, which was not an easy feat. His tiny fragile body was skeletal because it was unable to absorb any nutrients. Days turned into weeks without so much as an ounce gained. Their solution: a feeding tube called a gavage, a long tube that was threaded through his nose and down to his stomach so liquid food and supplements could be fed to him. What a sight this skeletal deformed-faced infant was. The trach kept him breathing, and the gavage tube kept him fed. While Hugh's medical team was able to keep him alive, there was a shared belief that he would never be able to talk. Years later when he acquired his medical records, he was surprised to see that he was labeled as "nonverbal and retarded." Apparently, the team felt this child would never develop intellectually. Believing he could not hear, he was also deemed "deaf." With life-threatening physical problems and such pessimistic predictions toward his future development, the deck of life was stacked against him. Even though all concerned struggled to keep him alive, many believed he would have been much better off had he died because none of them could envision a viable future for him. Collectively, it was believed he would most likely be institutionalized. There appeared to be very little hope among them that he could possibly lead any semblance of a normal life.

A few months later when Hugh was stabilized, he was released to the care of the state of Indiana and their foster care program.

An Angel Unaware

Across the White River from Riley Hospital for Children in one of the poorest and roughest sections of inner-city Indianapolis lived an elderly African American woman, Mrs. Lillian Collins. Barely five feet tall and weighing less than one hundred pounds, her home was a tiny run-down bungalow with constantly locked doors and windows and splintered wood floors that she shared with her birth daughters and various foster children. What Mrs. Collins lacked in material wealth, she was abundantly blessed with spiritual and emotional generosity. Her God-given calling was to care for the unwanted and sickly children no one else would take. In fact, Riley Hospital worked very closely with her by placing many of the "unwanted" in her hands. She devoted her life to these children no one else wanted then.

When Baby Hugh was six months old and finally strong enough, he was handed over to Mrs. Collins. For the next two years, he was the bottomless recipient of Mrs. Collins's and her biological daughters' unconditional love and devotion. It appeared they were all fighting for his life. There was so much more to his existence than feeding and cleaning him; that was the easy part. No one had prepared her for his very dominant, headstrong personality that steadily emerged. More and more, Mrs. Collins found herself dealing with his Irish stubbornness, hardheadedness, and ferocious temper tantrums. Now known simply as Hugh, he was confined to his crib, not out of meanness but for his own protection. The rough wood floors were badly splintered. Some of her other foster children were frightening at best and could not be trusted around her sickly charge. At that time, it was not known for certain if Hugh was deaf. They believed he was. Unable to communicate, he threw ferocious temper tantrums that Mrs. Collins placated by giving in to him, anything to keep him quiet! This only served to reinforce his behavior even more. Soon, the sickly toddler was the master ruler of his own fiefdom in the Collins's home by doing very little more than wielding his mighty temper.

In the two years Hugh lived with Mrs. Collins, foster mother and son grew to love each other as any biological bonded mother and son would. It was a bittersweet day when the state of Indiana found a home in which to place him. He was two and a half years old.

Chapter 2

God's Sovereignty in Motion
1933–1959

Somewhere in Rural Illinois (1933)

The late-night autumn weather had a biting chill to it, signaling the beginning of winter. Parked on the side of a flat dismal rural road somewhere in Illinois was an older car that towed a homemade trailer home. The gusts of wind periodically caused the trailer to veer one way or the other before it righted itself. Through a small covered window, the light of a lantern was barely detected.

Inside the trailer home was a family of four. Ray and Ruth Johnson, both early thirties, and their two children—Betty, ten years old, and her brother, Bobby, who was eight. The trailer home was fairly new. Prior, the family hitchhiked together, everywhere, so Ray could look for work. One time, a lady saw them standing by the side of the road with their thumbs out. She approached them with a large paper sack filled with shelled pecans and roasted yams. "You can stay in the shed if you want," she stated. Its wood floor was pine. "It's soft. Now lie down and go to sleep." Safe from the outside elements, the shed was their haven. The time they were provided enabled Ray to build the trailer home and somehow acquire a car to pull it.

Ray, a construction worker and tile layer, had a tremendous eye for detail. He was a good, very hardworking man who always provided well for his family even when circumstances were at their worst. Ruth, the granddaughter of a Swedish immigrant, was a God-fearing woman who loved the LORD and gave completely and selflessly for her husband and children. It was she who raised their children to depend on and obey Scripture and believe in grace by faith alone. Every night, she read from the Bible aloud to their family and encouraged the children to lead prayer time. The children knew their LORD was in all things and would never leave or forsake them.

The family huddled together, wearing as much clothing as possible for warmth while lying on top of strewn newspapers with one flimsy blanket to cover all of them. Under an old dress Ruth used as her pillow was her parents' family Bible. Four years into the Great Depression, like millions of other destitute Americans, they struggled to find work and food in order to keep the family together. They hadn't eaten in four days, and they were all suffering from hunger pangs. Ray and Ruth were engaged in a whispering argument.

"No," hissed Ruth. "I will not hear of it. We're a family, and we stay together no matter what."

Ray retorted, "But you don't understand. Winter is almost here. I need to find work. It makes sense to get you and the children settled, and I can send you money for food."

"I said no. I will not—"

"Lower your voice. You'll wake the—"

Betty let out a shriek. "You hurt Dolly. Look what you did!" Betty shoved her brother over as hard as she could. Bobby let out a cry and shoved her back.

Dolly was Betty's Raggedy Anne doll, the one that never left her side. Betty took as loving care of Dolly as any mother would her own child. There was a small tear in Dolly's leg, and some sawdust stuffing fell out and onto the blanket.

"Children! Stop it at once!" demanded Ruth. Both children were whimpering.

Ray sternly said, "Do as your mother says. Right now."

"I'm hungry," cried Bobby. "Do we have to skip another meal?"

"I know, Honey," replied Ruth. "We're not skipping a meal. We're just postponing one for a little bit longer."

Ruth changed the subject. She turned toward Betty. "Honey, let's give Dolly to Daddy so he can fix her up." Ruth gently took the doll from Betty and handed it to Ray. She eyed the small amount of sawdust on the blanket as if it was gold. She nudged Ray to look. He nodded.

"Honey, sit still. Let me get the sawdust from your blanket." Carefully, she scooped the sawdust from the blanket into her hand as if it was gold dust. It was about a tablespoon.

They nodded their heads.

Ruth read aloud, "The LORD fed them by dropping manna from heaven. It wasn't the food they wanted, but it was what they needed in order to survive. Our LORD knows how hungry we are, and we have to trust in Him to provide for us. Do you trust Him?"

The children both nodded.

"Mommy," piped in Betty, "let's pray and tell Jesus how hungry we are."

Ruth replied, "First, let's read what the Bible says about the LORD taking care of our needs."

Ruth opened the Bible to Psalm 81:10. She gathered the children close to her. Ray continued to fix Dolly's tear.

"I am the LORD thy God, which brought thee out of the land of Egypt; open thy mouth wide, and I will fill it." Ruth continued with the Psalm. The children were quieted.

"Dear LORD in heaven, we love you and ask that you forgive us for our trespasses as we forgive others for theirs against us. You know our situation. Please help Daddy find work. We hold you to your promises to meet our needs. We are very hungry, LORD. We ask that you provide for us during these terrible times. No matter what, we love you and trust in you. Amen."

"Amen," they whispered collectively.

"The LORD will take care of us in His own good time. Remember, children, God's timing is perfect. Through this trial we are going through, he is preparing us for things that are to come in our lives later on, and He is teaching us patience while building out faith. Keep your eyes upon

Jesus and not our problems." Ruth gently closed the Bible with careful reverence.

Under Betty's towel that made do as her pillow was a well-worn copy of *Little Women* by Louisa May Alcott, a gift from her grandmother. This was her favorite book and one she read over and over.

"Are you reading that book again, Honey? Why, you're going to read the words right off its pages." Ruth paused. "Do you still want to be just like Jo when you grow up?"

Betty brightened up. "Yes, I'm going to have lots of children no one else wants, just like her. Only, I'm going to have girls too."

"I know you will. You're going to be a wonderful mother someday." Ruth glanced at her husband.

Ray handed Dolly back to Betty. She scowled. "How come her legs are different, Daddy?"

"I removed the sawdust from both legs and replaced it with shredded newspaper, Sweetheart. That way, the legs look the same."

Betty wasn't certain. She inspected Dolly from head to toe. Finally, she said, "I'll just have to love her even more now that she's a little different."

"Okay, children, let's get back to bed," said Ray. The couple hugged their children good night and got them settled in.

The children huddled down together, and within moments, they were sound asleep. Ray and Ruth lay next to them, clinging to each other.

"Honey," whispered Ray, "we barely have enough gas to go anywhere. Tomorrow, I will walk into the field and see what I can find."

"Perhaps there are some berries or plants somewhere we missed. Betty likes those. Let's pray for some meat. Now that we have some sawdust, we can extend what little we find. Remember, Bobby won't eat skunk or opossum."

In a soft whisper barely heard, Ruth began to pray.

Then He took the five loaves and the two fishes,
and looking up to heaven, He blessed them and broke them and
gave to the disciples to set before the multitudes.

—Luke 9:16

Shantytown

By the time Ray finally found enough work to keep his family together, the rest of Dolly was stuffed with shredded newspapers, her sawdust being put to many uses. Her ever-changing physique made Betty cling to her even more.

After numerous and frequent moves, many under barely survivable conditions, Ray settled his family into a shantytown that was filled with an amazing eclectic group of people. Traveling salesmen, tradesmen, oil riggers, migrants, carnival workers, and gypsies called it home. Many of the improvised homes were made from cardboard or some other flimsy material that could be used to create a temporary shelter. Very few others, like the Johnsons, had homemade trailers.

Life around the camp was never dull. Carnival workers were abundant, and their outlandish garb and colorful stories were wildly entertaining. Madonna, a carnival dancer who was Betty's age, was attending the same correspondence school as Betty was for her education. Best friends, the girls studied together nightly, and both girls earned their diplomas. In spite of the times and their difficult surroundings, it was a time of bonding, and more often than not, the focus was not the hardship of the times but on each other.

Ray and Ruth worked hard to make Betty and Bobby feel special during these times of extreme hardship. Their reward was that both children reached out to others, so they too felt special. It wasn't long before Betty fell in love with a fragile tiny little crippled gypsy baby named Maria. In the campfire light where everyone gathered at night for warmth and stories, Betty could see her smiling back at her. The baby's matted long black hair only enhanced her dark mahogany skin and deep melancholy eyes, the kind that always seem to brim with tears. She was a very well-loved, happy little girl who delighted in her times with Betty.

Then there was the little African American boy named Joey who was so filled with joy he was contagious. His family lived in a dilapidated old cabin in various stages of decay a short way from the camp. Almost nightly, Betty could see Joey's mother drop mounds of laundry into boiling water in exchange for a meager pittance from anyone who could afford this luxury. Joey and his little brother delighted in dressing up in the laundry that arrived in huge baskets until their mother caught them one night and chased them all around camp with her broom.

Migrant worker families lived together in their old beater cars. It was obvious they were in extreme poverty, but their family units were so strong and loving they couldn't help but inspire others around them.

Betty remembers these difficult times with joy, not bitterness or anger. She learned early to love people from all walks of life and found herself praying for each of them. No matter what their situation, or how bad it was, the LORD always provided. Sometimes His timing stretched beyond their patience, but He never let them down. Betty, especially, leaned on the LORD from a very early age. Looking back, she sees how God was preparing her for a difficult but blessed, uncharted journey filled with heartbreak, disappointments, and, above all, miracles, that was to become her future. Still, no matter what, the Johnsons had a sense of peace and joy in their midst they could not deny. They had dignity. Others saw it too and often mentioned it.

What About Bob? (1933)

A Galesburg, Illinois, native, Bob's parents met during World War I. Bob's father was in the army, and his mother was a Red Cross nurse.

Bob's devout Catholic family was also a very loving and close family. He had two younger brothers and a sister, and they all cared for one another deeply. But of the four children, it was Bob who was exceptionally close to his father.

Bob's father was much admired in his community, and no one admired him more than his eldest son. From early on, he made it his personal mission to emulate his father's very high standards. Tragically, when Bob was only twelve, his father was killed in an automobile accident. Immediately, he became the man of the house and the keeper of his father's legend. Nothing pleased him more than to be told he was just like his father.

Then Pearl Harbor was attacked. Like thousands of other heroic young men, Bob left college at an early age to serve his country. He enlisted in the U.S. Army Air Corps as a mechanic where he served for the next five years. It was shortly after he returned from the war when he met his future bride.

A Very Special Love Story

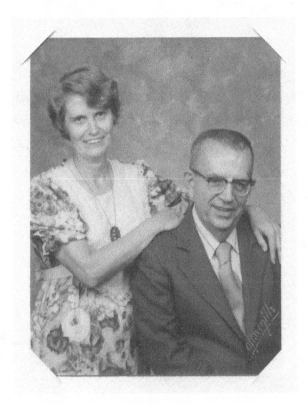

Betty Johnson Smith and Bob Smith

Husbands, love your wives,
As Christ loved the church
And gave himself up for her, that he might sanctify her,
Having cleansed her by the washing of water with the word,
So that he might present the church to himself in splendor,
Without spot or wrinkle or any such thing,
That she might be holy and without blemish.
In the same way husbands should love their wives
as their own bodies.
He who loves his wife loves himself.
For no one ever hated his own flesh,
But nourishes and cherishes it,
Just as Christ does the church…

—Ephesians 5:25–33

Chapter 3

Song of Solomon
1950

For lo,
The winter is past,
The rain is over and gone;
The flowers appear on the earth;
The time of the singing of birds is come,
And the voice of the turtle
Is heard in our land.

—Song of Solomon 2:11–12:7

A Very Special Love Story

Betty attended Northwestern University in Chicago and married at a young age. Almost one year later, their son, Andrew, was born. Her dream of having a family of her own was off to an early start.

What Betty did not know until it was too late, her husband had been diagnosed with tuberculosis. Not only did his illness threaten the health of his young wife and son but she was completely in the dark that her husband's illness would soon kill him.

By accident, she found out that her husband was seriously ill. He had hidden the medical evidence of his terminal illness in the back of his underwear drawer, where she found it. After she had confronted him with it, he admitted he had kept this devastating news from her on purpose because he feared, if she knew, she would take their son and leave him. Although she never would have left him, she was frightened. By the time she found out, her husband had only a few more weeks to live. There was little, if any, time to prepare for the fact that she was soon going to be a widow with a young son she was going to have to raise on her own.

A talented seamstress, Betty found work in nearby Crystal Lake at Spic and Span Dry Cleaners, where she was hired to do alterations. Unable to afford day care for Andrew, she carried him on the commuter train to work every workday. Packed in her carryall bag filled with her son's necessities and their lunches was her small pocket Bible. Inside the crowded train, she would often sit quietly and read scriptures in a very soft voice to her son.

Meanwhile, Andrew was happily ensconced in the back office at the dry cleaners where Betty and Mrs. Stein constantly doted on him.

By then, Mrs. Stein was looking for someone to help manage her business, a business she took much pride in because of her faithful clientele. She had very strong bonds with all of them, and she wanted her employees to be as well-liked as she was. She wouldn't hire just anybody.

> *You are altogether beautiful*
> *My love*
> *There is no flaw in you.*
>
> —Song of Solomon 4:7

Love at First Sight—Almost

Shortly after Betty began working at the dry-cleaning store, Mrs. Stein hired a handsome, very affable young man who had served in the war whom she liked immediately. His name was Bob Smith.

From the first time Bob saw Betty hard at work at her sewing machine, he was completely taken by her. Diligently, he had been praying for a godly woman to be his wife and the mother of the large family he longed for, and in that moment, he believed he had found her. Immediately, he had noticed that there was something special about her. Besides being a fresh and natural beauty, there was a sense of peace and calm about her he couldn't help but notice. In that moment, she was focused on her job at hand and didn't notice the handsome man standing in front of her, staring at her. She lifted her head for a polite hello when Mrs. Stein introduced them; then she went right back to her task at hand.

Almost immediately, Bob's hopes were dashed. One step inside the back office, he stopped in his tracks. Andrew was happily playing with some toys his mother had brought to amuse him. He immediately assumed she must be married. When Andrew looked up at Bob and smiled, his heart sank.

As the days and weeks passed by, Betty was far too focused on her job to take much notice of Bob other than having to talk to him about work. All that was on her mind other than her work was Andrew.

At lunch when the store was closed, Betty would go to the back office where she and Andrew ate their lunches together. It wasn't quite spring yet, so it was too chilly to spend lunchtime outside, so they played on the floor and laughed and laughed.

Bob's hopes were suddenly raised one day when he was in the back office. Mrs. Stein walked in and noticing his longing look at Andrew, she said, "What a pity Betty lost her husband. He's such a beautiful, sweet-natured little boy. She's doing a wonderful job caring for him. I hate to see her having to struggle so much."

Standing alone in the office, Bob's heart was overwhelmed. He adored Andrew, and he was completely captivated by his mother. Next to him on the table was Andrew's carryall bag. On top of its contents was Betty's pocket Bible. In that exact moment, he knew he had found the woman who was meant to be his wife. All he had to do was persuade her.

***

As soon as the winter weather finally turned into springtime, Bob gathered up his courage to ask Betty if she and Andrew would join him for lunch, and he was nervous. Although he hesitated, he convinced her that the warm, fresh air after such a long winter would do her good.

"Well, I have Andrew, you know," she said hesitantly.

"Why, he's the most important guest of all, after his beautiful mother, of course," Bob cooed in his charming voice.

Betty choked back laughter at the almost-smarmy remark. For the first time, Bob saw her laugh, and it touched his soul.

Across the street from the store was an outdoor café that was soon filled to capacity. Bob's sandwich remained untouched as he watched Betty lovingly share her sandwich with her son.

Bob couldn't contain himself another moment. He leaned over and said, "Betty, I'm going to marry you."

Betty did a double take. "What?"

He had her full attention. "Betty, from the first moment I saw you, you took my breath away. When I went to the back office and saw Andrew, I was crushed. I thought you were married. Later on, Mrs. Stein told me you were a widow. I'm so sorry for your loss, Betty." She nodded. "A few days later, I saw your pocket Bible in your carryall. That's when I knew my prayers were answered."

"Oh, Bob, how sweet of you. Thank you. But my life is all about Andrew now. Besides, I'm still not over my husband's death."

"I see your struggles, Betty. You're a wonderful mother. I've been praying for a lovely, godly woman to be my wife and the mother to my children."

Betty was speechless. Her eyes locked with Bob. Slowly, she considered this very well could be the man for her and Andrew.

> *I have found the one*
> *Whom my soul loves.*
>
> —Song of Solomon 3:4

A Summertime Proposal

Several weeks later, Betty sat in Bob's large dark green sedan, waiting patiently for Bob to return with their ice cream. It was a hot and humid summer night. The outdoor area was packed with families and teenagers and friends who all gulped down their ice cream treats.

Andrew was happily amused in the back car seat. The bright neon lights from the ice cream parlor danced happily across the windshield, filling the car with a rainbow of colors, and he was captivated. Bob hurried out of the store, opened the driver's door, and handed Betty her chocolate cone. He then reached over the seat to hand Andrew his cone.

Betty was mortified. "Oh, dear, I think it would be much better if Andrew's ice cream was in a cup. Maybe we should eat outside."

"You worry too much, Betty. Andrew has to learn to eat a cone sometime, right, little fella?" Bob chuckled.

"I can't look." Betty cringed.

"Relax. It's all washable." Bob settled in behind the wheel. He thought for a moment before saying, "Betty, have you thought anymore about what I said to you a few weeks ago?"

Andrew let out a cry as the cone fell to the floor, leaving a partial scoop of the ice cream in his lap. The rest of it was smeared all over the car seat and window.

"Oh no!" gasped Betty.

"He's washable too." Bob laughed. After a moment, he turned serious. "Betty, look at me." She turned toward him. "I love you. I have loved you from the first moment I saw you. I want nothing more than to be your husband and Andrew's father. Just think. You, me, Andrew, and lots more children raised for the LORD."

Bob and Betty stared into each other's eyes. They were both still. A moment passed before he quietly said, "Betty, will you marry me?"

Betty pondered his words to her. In a quiet, very soft voice, Betty answered him, "Yes." They embraced and kissed.

Andrew let out a delighted squeal, picked up the blob of ice cream from his lap, and threw it at them, hitting both their faces.

"I guess we just got Andrew's seal of approval." Bob laughed. Betty let out a laugh.

Rise up, my love
My fair one
And come away with me.

—Song of Solomon 2:10

A Destiny Is Sealed

God's hand was apparent from the very beginning in the lives of Bob and Betty. She was the most beautiful bride. Even their pastor commented on her elegance and grace. Her floor-length white dress with its train and long flowing veil created a vision of awe in the small chapel. With her handsome groom by her side and with family and friends looking on, they were pronounced husband and wife.

As soon as they walked down the outside steps, their excited guests hailed them with rice, an age-old tradition that was believed to bring wealth and prosperity to the couple and the assurance of fertility. Everyone knew Bob and Betty's desire was to raise a large family for their LORD.

Covered in rice and laughing, the excited newlyweds rushed to Bob's green sedan and hopped inside. They both turned and waved to their guests who viewed them through the back windshield with "Just Married" painted on it, followed by a noisy bunch of tin cans tied to the bumper with twine.

Thus began their new life as husband and wife. For Andrew, it was more than that; he now had a father who loved him as his own. Foremost on all their minds was starting a new family.

Chapter 4

God's Plans Are Not Our Plans
1959

In All Your Ways, Acknowledge Him

The noisy clanking bustle of the hospital breakfast time intruded into Betty's now-forgotten dream. Groggily, her eyes began to flutter open. Betty grimaced from a sudden jolt of pain that slowly began to subside. Protectively, her hand rested on her very painful stitches-filled abdomen. In small flashes, she remembered the rush to the hospital and into emergency surgery, with Bob holding her hand until he could go no farther. A faint smile came to her face. She had just given birth. Was it a boy or a girl? She couldn't wait to find out.

What caught her attention next was the fragrance of the beautiful red roses in a vase next to her Bible on the nightstand, a gift from her husband and son, Bob and Andrew. She turned toward the nightstand and breathed in the heavenly aroma as the roses began to come into focus.

Slightly more alert, Betty glanced around as best she could from her prone position. The pale blue walls of her hospital room brought comfort. On the wall next to her bed was a single portrait, a painting of Jesus.

Betty smiled. "LORD," she murmured softly to herself, "I feel your presence. Thank you." She desperately wanted her newborn in her arms.

Betty began to realize she was not alone. She could hear a hushed conversation. Turning toward the voices, she blinked against the bright sunlight that filtered through the curtain room divider. In silhouette, she saw the nurse leaning over another patient in the bed next to hers. They were talking softly.

The woman was saying, "Is the woman next to me all right? She's been sleeping for nearly twenty-four hours."

The nurse practically whispered her reply, "She had emergency childbirth surgery two days ago. We didn't think she would make it."

"Oh my goodness," replied the faceless voice. "I hope she'll be all right. What about her baby?"

"It is going to be very difficult for her when she wakes up. Her baby boy passed away early this morning. This is the eleventh child she has lost."

"Oh, dear God! What can I do?" gasped the patient.

"Pray for her," said the nurse.

Betty was stunned. It took her a moment to grasp what she just heard. *Two days?* She had been sleeping for two entire days? Her *son?* She had a son? No, they weren't talking about *her* son. Her baby was born by caesarean section, and she could see him any moment now. Slowly, the sorrow sank in. Her eyes welled with tears as what she feared the most was now her reality. Yes, it was her baby who was gone. His name was Joseph. She turned back toward the roses and began to pray. "Thank you, LORD, for the beauty and scent of these roses. Your presence is in all things." She closed her eyes and let the sobs come. The tears roll down her face.

Moments later, Andrew, who was now thirteen years old, and Bob walked in and stood by Betty's bedside. She looked into Bob's and Andrew's eyes. All she could see was their heartbreak. The three of them remained silent as Bob reached over and took his wife's hand in his.

"Joseph is gone," cried Betty, half asking, half telling.

Bob nodded then bowed his head, holding the hands of Betty and Andrew. Betty's own life had been seriously jeopardized, and she was still extremely weak from her own profuse blood loss. "Thank you, LORD Jesus, for the eight months Betty was able to carry our son, Joseph Wendall Smith, under her heart. Please give Betty strength and healing. We know your plans are bigger than our plans. We now rejoice that our precious son is with you now and forever. Amen."

A short while later, Betty was taken to a private room. A friend had driven Andrew home so Bob could remain by his wife's side. How sweet it was of her son to want to be there when she woke up. He had always insisted on being beside her through each of their losses. Sometimes she worried about him, but he had always insisted he wouldn't have it any other way. These losses weren't just hers; they were Bob's and Andrew's as well. A nurse came in and stuck a syringe into her IV. She fell back asleep.

Proverbs 3:5—"Trust in the LORD"

Hours later, Betty was sitting upright, with her Bible open to Proverbs 3:5 on her lap: "Trust in the Lord with all your heart and lean not unto thine own understanding."

Betty stared blankly at the wall; her dinner tray was pushed aside, untouched. Bob sat next to her, holding her hand. Silently, they comforted each other as they dealt with the loss of their newborn son. Even with their deep faith and trust in the LORD, their loss was unbearably heartbreaking. Neither one of them heard Dr. Jeffries, their obstetrician, enter the room.

Dr. Jeffries approached Betty's bed. His normal rather curt bedside manner was temporarily put aside, and it was obvious that he was as bereft as they were. Bob and Betty gave him their attention.

"Mr. and Mrs. Smith, I cannot find the words to tell you how very sorry I am about Joseph. I must tell you both I share in your great sadness," Dr. Jeffries stated sadly with tears in his own eyes. In a moment, he reverted back to being a doctor.

"I'll get to the point. As your obstetrician, I cannot allow you to get pregnant again. I spent much of this afternoon reviewing your case. Your emotional and psychological health are just as much at risk now as your physical health is. I'm so sorry." Dr. Jeffries paused. "Will you be willing to adopt?" he asked.

Bob and Betty took in the long-overdue news. They both nodded in agreement.

"If Joseph was meant to be the earthly adopted father of Jesus, then adoption is good enough for us," Bob quietly replied.

Dr. Jeffries went on, "Adoption can be a very long and tedious process. Unless—"

Through her tears, Betty continued the sentence from where he left off. "Unless...we take in children, special children, rejected children, imperfect children, waiting children, children no one else wants. The children the LORD intended, just for us."

As He was with Sarah and Abraham, the LORD had a plan.

A person plans his course,
But the Lord directs his steps.

—Proverbs 16:9

Chapter 5

Let the Journey Begin
1961–1965

Holding Fast to His Ways

Situated on a lovely tree-lined street with large grass yards in Champaign, Illinois, was the modest, well-kept home of the Smith family. Two years had gone by since the passing of Joseph, but Betty and Bob continued their steady pursuit of prayer and adoption. The sorrow of their marriage was that they lost every single one of their eleven pregnancies from miscarriages, stillbirths, and dying shortly after birth. It was only inevitable that the Smiths' obstetrician would forbid another pregnancy.

There were eleven lost lives in all. Betty could not help her times of bitterness. "How could God do this?" she often cried. Bob felt differently. He accepted it all without question. Dr. Jeffries encouraged them not to dwell on their losses or to lose hope. He told them they would someday have a large family. He didn't know how or why; he just knew.

The Smiths did not go into the adoption journey blindly. Bob, Betty, and Andrew faithfully prayed without ceasing. Betty read every book and article on adoption and learned everything she could about the process. They had the support of their parish priest, their obstetrician, and friends. But the most difficult of all was the lack of response from the numerous letters she sent out. It was a waiting game that would have tried the patience of the saintliest of saints. During their ceaseless praying, Bob often quoted Job 23:11: "My foot has held fast to His steps; I have kept His way and not turned aside."

One Saturday afternoon, Betty sat at the kitchen table staring pensively at the open adoption catalogs and letters she had just written that were stacked next to her Bible.

"Hi, Mom!" Andrew burst through the door. His baseball uniform was covered in dirt and mud. At the kitchen sink, he gulped a large glass of water.

"How did the game go, Honey?" Betty inquired. "Where's your dad?"

"We won. Dad's cleaning up." Andrew approached the table. "Still writing letters, Mom? It's been two years."

Betty remained silent. Andrew leaned over and gave her a hug. "Don't give up, Mom. I pray every night for a brother or a sister."

"We all do, Honey." Betty paused. "We are being tested. I won't stop writing until the LORD tells me to."

Bob came through the kitchen, fresh from his shower. He leaned over the table and kissed Betty.

Bob said, "It was just on the news that President Kennedy announced that there are real problems in South Vietnam and that we are going to send in—"

The wall phone rang, stopping Bob midsentence. He turned and picked up the phone. "Hello?" He paused. "Yes, this is he." Pause. "A boy? How old? Four?"

Betty jumped up. Excited, she and Andrew gathered close to the phone so they could hear.

"His name is Billy? Yes, we can be there first thing tomorrow morning. What time?"

Bob hung up the phone and hugged his wife and son. They hugged one another excitedly.

Bob prayed. "Thank you, LORD, for blessing us with our new son, Billy. Please bless our home and our family when he joins us. Please let us be the best parents and family possible for our new son."

"Amen," they chorused together as Betty wiped away her tears.

***

The arrival of Billy into the Smith family was met with such a flurry of happiness and excitement that none of them fully grasped the early warning signs that something was seriously amiss with their new son. No matter how hard any of them tried, Billy displayed an early aversion to touch and physical affection. One moment, he would be unresponsive, and the next, he would have an angry, unprovoked, and frightening outburst. Little was known about his background, so the Smiths dealt with their new child in the best way they knew how, by treating him with love and praying for him.

Their time alone as a family with their new son was short-lived. Within one year of Billy's adoption, four other children of different ages and challenges and races immediately began to follow. First was Edwin who was nine years old. Emotionally, he was a blah child. It appeared he was incapable of displaying any emotions. Tragically, Edwin was the only survivor out of his entire family that was killed in a terrible house fire. The only reason he survived was because his father threw him out of the attic window in order to save him from the burning flames. Nearly every bone in his body was broken on impact. Although his bones mended, his psyche did not. After countless surgeries, his body was filled with painful bone chips that plagued him day and night. In chronic pain, he was kept heavily medicated. He would hang his head, his hair in his eyes, and respond to very little, if at all. He never argued and always did as he was asked. But what bothered them the most was that he would not make eye contact with any of them. Edwin was a heartbreaking challenge, but Bob and Betty loved and prayed for him, knowing that would pay off in the long run, but for now, there was no change.

Peter, a dark-skinned Hopi Indian came to them next, not quite a year old. He had already been adopted, but his migrant adoptive parents could no longer care for him financially. When he arrived at the Smiths' home less than a year after Edwin, he was sick with a severe case of rickets, his stomach was bloated from malnourishment, and there were bald spots all over his head. Adding to the problem, he had only been spoken to in Spanish, a language the Smiths did not know. Thus, communication was a daily struggle.

Four Years Later

As Bob and Betty moved forward with their growing family, never a day went by that she didn't thank the LORD for the wonderful God-fearing, patient husband she was given. Evident to everyone was theirs was a God-ordained match. Every single day, she was amazed at how well the LORD had prepared them both very early on for His plans for their lives.

"Both of us grew up with very little. I learned how to cook and how to make a penny spread as far as it would go. I sewed a lot and made everyone's clothes," she reminisced. "Bob had suffered tremendous losses, and he became the man of his family very early on."

Bob was excellent about doing whatever needed to be done around the house even though, as an engineer for Magnavox, it was required that he travel quite a bit. He was an excellent husband, father, and provider and never quibbled about taking on extra work as a bookkeeper and tax preparer for a good number of clientele. He was as hands on with the children as Betty was when he was home. What she was most thankful for was that he considered Andrew to be as much his son as hers. "Not all men want to take on another man's child," recalled Betty. Bob was different from the very beginning. He wanted to be Andrew's father as much as he wanted to be Betty's husband. "He was wonderful." It was their teamwork that allowed them to pursue the large family they dreamed about from the very beginning.

An Unexpected Arrival (1965)

Angel was a completely unexpected arrival into the lives of the Smith family. Her biological parents had been involved in a head-on collision that killed the father on impact and left Angel's heavily pregnant mother fighting for her life. Knowing she wouldn't survive the birth of her precious infant, the mother's last act of courage was to choose her baby's adopted parents out of a catalog. She chose the Smiths.

The biological mother died in childbirth. Horrified by her tragic plight, the Smiths didn't hesitate to take her precious newborn into their family. Of Argentinian descent, Angel, as they named her, was only three days old when she arrived at their home a restless, temperamental newborn who somehow knew she had suffered a tragedy of insurmountable proportions.

No sooner than Betty had gotten Angel settled in, Bob arrived home unexpectedly early. His crushed demeanor immediately alerted Betty.

"Honey, you're home early," Betty said.

Bob seated himself at the kitchen table without saying a word. Betty quietly joined him.

"Is something wrong?" Betty asked quietly.

Bob waited a moment before telling her the unwanted news. "I lost my job today."

"What?" Betty felt sickened. Bob was an engineer for Magnavox, and back in those days, in the sixties, an employee joined a company for life because your career was an extension of your family. While their children were deemed foster children, the state helped with medical expenses, and they continued to help when and if they became permanent foster children. Magnavox had graciously agreed to pick up all the medical expenses of their growing family, and their expenses were growing as fast as their family. Only after their children were legally adopted were they completely on their own, and even then, Magnavox picked up their expenses. With Bob's job loss, there was no longer any medical coverage. With a trembling voice, Betty asked her husband, "Why? What happened? Were you fired?"

Bob shook his head. "No. The engineering division is being transferred to Mexico. I was offered the job, but I won't uproot you and the children. I'll have to find another job."

Betty was totally deflated. "What are we going to do? We're in the middle of adopting Angel. We can't adopt her now. The judge will never allow us to take her if you don't have a job. What about the other children? We have so much—"

"Betty," Bob quieted his wife, "let's allow the LORD to take care of this. We'll just have to cut back on every unnecessary medical expense and pray that we don't have any emergencies. In the meantime, I'll be looking for a new job."

That evening, Bob and Betty began their ceaseless prayers for provision, protection, and guidance for a new job for Bob.

Judge Lubarsky

Judge Lubarsky looked Bob and Betty straight into their eyes. He could see a glimmer of unease, but they were the same family whose adoptions he had been tending to for years now.

"I have all the faith in the world in you, Mr. and Mrs. Smith. You'll be just fine. I've been processing your adoptions from the beginning, and I'm not going to take Angel away from you. Your unemployment, I'm certain, is temporary. I am granting you full custody of your new daughter, Angel."

Thankfully, Bob's unemployment was short-lived. After three months of traveling to try and find work, Magnavox called and offered him his old job back. Relocating the engineering department to Mexico had not worked out.

The Blessings Keep on Coming

Their next daughter, Susie, was barely one year old when she was placed in an orphanage to die, not to live, and it was God's hand that led her to the Smiths. A dear friend of Betty who ran the orphanage called her one night, desperate for help. The flu was going around, and most of her caregivers had called in sick, and now even some of the babies were sick. Bob agreed to take care of the household so Betty could help out. During the rounds of changing diapers and feedings, she leaned into Susie's crib and almost reeled from the shock. Cerebral palsy caused her body to be as stiff as a board. Tape covered her eyes because she was going blind.

"I knew at once that God had a plan for this beautiful baby," remembered Betty.

Betty reached in to touch this traumatized child. Susie grabbed her finger and wouldn't let go. It was a moment of understanding for Betty, knowing that, if she didn't take this helpless child, she wouldn't survive. As soon as she arrived home, she told Bob about her. That night, they knelt beside their bed and prayed together for guidance. A few days later, Susie was in their arms. There was more yet to come for Susie. It was discovered she had a serious congenital heart condition that if not corrected, soon she would die.

Susie seemed to weather her storms with little trauma, but the one thing that completely baffled Bob and Betty was that she became fixated on light bulbs. She stared and stared at them endlessly. It got to the point where lights couldn't be turned on anywhere near her. Edwin, their first adopted son after Billy, solved the riddle, and his explanation shook them to their very core. "Don't you know that when you're in a children's home, at night in the nursery, a light bulb is sort of like your mom," he said.

Andrew Jerome Smith

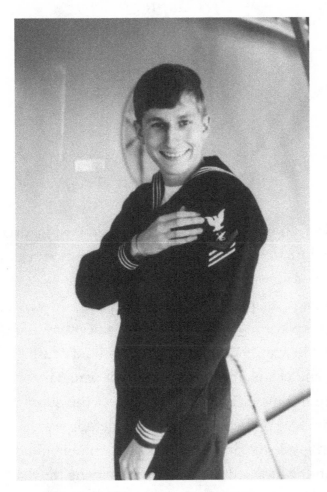

Andrew joins the navy.

Chapter 6

The Heartbreak Kid

A Troubled Family (1965)

Betty looked out the kitchen window while drying the dishes, lost in worried thought. Billy was now eight years old and was outside playing alone. Queenie, the family Queensland shepherd, was sniffing along the fence. Even alone, his playing was rough, and his demeanor was mean. He couldn't be with the other children without causing trouble, upset, and chaos. In spite of constant parental corrections, love, punishment, and ongoing prayer, he simply refused to respond. His behavior was only getting worse, and the tension inside the Smith home was becoming unbearable.

Andrew walked in the kitchen carrying the daily newspaper. "Do you need any help, Mom?" he asked.

"No, thank you, Honey. I'm almost done." Betty stopped drying the dishes and looked out the window at what was once a beautiful tree. "I wonder what is going on with that poor tree? It looks awful."

Andrew stood next to Betty. "I have no idea. It's been like that for a while." Andrew changed the subject. "It said on the news that the Civil Rights Act is already in motion."

Betty shook her head then turned her attention back to the dishes. "Thank God for that. I can't wait for this whole thing to settle…" Betty opened the knife drawer and stopped midsentence.

"Andrew, the utility knife is missing. Where could it have possibly gone? I didn't use it this morning," Betty said.

"I don't know," Andrew replied, still staring at the tree.

An awful *thud* came from the street, followed by the sound of squealing brakes. The woman driver bolted out of the car, screaming.

"No! Oh God, no!"

Andrew bolted out the kitchen side door and onto the street as Betty rushed into the family room. Safe and sound, Edwin, Peter, Susie, and Angel were all together in front of the television.

Betty turned and rushed out the kitchen door. Over the fence, she yelled. "Billy! Billy!" Betty screamed. "Get in the house. Now!"

Andrew's Broken Heart

Andrew huddled in front of the car, completely bloodied.

Before anyone could stop her, Betty was standing next to her son. Her hands flew to her mouth as she let out a scream.

"No! Oh my God, no!"

Queenie was badly mangled and bleeding heavily. Andrew tried to shield their dying pet from his mother's eyes, but it was too late. He gently picked up the seventy-pound dog and cradled her in his arms as she took her last breath. Together, Andrew and Betty sobbed over their beloved pet while Queenie's blood dripped down both of them.

"How could this happen?" Betty sobbed. Andrew noticed the side gate to their yard was wide open.

"The gate is open. That's how she got out." Andrew started to sob.

Quelling her own emotions, Betty tried to comfort her son. Queenie was his dog ever since he rescued her as a pup from a garbage can. They were inseparable.

Wiping her eyes, Betty rushed through the gate and closed it behind her. The padlock that was kept on the gate was unlocked. Someone had to have done that.

A tearful crowd had formed. Someone offered a couple of towels that Andrew gratefully accepted.

Andrew carried Queenie into the yard and gently laid her on the ground. Billy let out a laugh. Andrew lunged right for Billy, and the two embroiled themselves in a fight. In seconds, they were both on the ground. Andrew was on top, and he was struggling to get something out of Billy's hand.

"You did this! You killed Queenie!" he screamed.

"Stop it! Stop it at once, you two!" Betty yelled.

Andrew stood, holding the missing utility knife he had wriggled out of Billy's hand. Mixed with Queenie's blood was now his own, dripping from a cut in his hand. Billy lay on the ground, laughing with a maniacal fervor.

"Mom," said Andrew, shaking, "look at the tree. He's been peeling the bark off of it!"

"Don't worry about that right now. Get in the bathroom and get your hand washed and bandaged. Oh, I wish your father was home," Betty agonized.

"I have to bury Queenie first," Andrew replied.

Billy let out a mocking sound. Andrew turned and lunged for Billy and yanked him to his feet.

"Stop it!" shouted Betty. Billy just smirked at both of them. Betty was close to losing her temper. "Go to your room. Your father will deal with you when he gets home. Now!"

Mr. Rogers, their next-door neighbor, came through the side gate. He looked at Andrew's cut hand. "You get inside and take care of that hand like your mother says. I'll get Queenie buried for you."

"Oh, Mr. Rogers, I don't know how to thank you. Bob won't be home until tonight," Betty cried.

"That's all right. You go take care of your son while I take care of this." He paused for a moment. "I'm so sorry, Mrs. Smith, Andrew."

Billy sauntered off without a care in the world. Betty and Andrew headed toward the front bathroom to tend to his knife cut. A loud *crash* turned their heads. Betty's curio cabinet that was filled with precious family heirlooms lay shattered across the hallway floor. When she realized what she was looking at, all she could do was stand there and cry.

In seconds, Andrew was by her side with his hand heavily bandaged. He grabbed his mother's elbow and guided her into the kitchen where she sat down at the table crying uncontrollably. Andrew stood beside her, so angry his face was flushed a deep red.

Andrew flew into a rage. "I hate him! How much longer are you and Dad going to keep letting him get away with this?"

"Andrew"—Betty gulped—"please don't hate him. I know he's terrible and something has to be done, but I don't know what. Your father and I are going to have a talk as soon as he gets home."

Betty was barely able to get through dinner that evening. Andrew was in pain and in mourning for his dog and didn't touch his food. He was glaring at Billy who didn't seem to care. The rest of the children were unusually quiet and just picking at their food. With Bob traveling, the burden was hers alone until he got home. Hours past her bedtime, Betty was still waiting for her husband.

While she counted the hours, she sat on the side of their bed crying—crying for Queenie, crying for Andrew, crying for Billy, and crying for her entire family. She longed for her husband's arms around her.

At two in the morning, Betty heard the sound of the car pulling into the garage. Bob was home. She dried her eyes and tried to make herself presentable. He wasn't used to finding his wife awake so late at night.

No sooner did he walk into their bedroom with a very perplexed look on his face as Betty burst into tears again.

He held and comforted her as she sobbed out the entire story.

***

Late that afternoon, Billy and Andrew were in their rooms, and the rest of the family was sitting in the family room. It had been a long day, and the tension was thick. The television was off, and the children were subdued. Bob and Betty sat on the couch, holding hands, quietly praying for guidance when the doorbell rang.

Bob got up to answer it. Marion Brown, Billy's social worker, entered with a dark look of concern on her face. She took one look at Betty, who was now standing next to Bob, tense and near tears.

"Oh dear," Marion sighed. "I'm so sorry it's so late. I had so much to do after I got your call this morning."

The trio entered the formal dining room and sat down at the table.

"On my way over here, I did a lot of thinking about your situation with Billy. This situation is only getting worse. We all know this cannot be allowed to go on anymore." She paused. "Have you eaten dinner yet?"

Bob and Betty shook their heads no.

"I'd like to suggest that you take the family out for dinner. I need to spend some time alone with Billy so I can assess him. That should take about two hours."

"That's fine," said Bob. "Let's get the kids ready, and we will leave."

Bob left the dining room and called Andrew. Betty and the social worker talked quietly for a few moments before she gathered the children.

An Unsettling Dinner

Even with the Civil Rights Bill in effect, it was still unheard of to see white parents with children of mixed races and physical challenges inside a white establishment. As soon as Bob and Betty ushered their eclectic family into the busy family-style restaurant, the room came to a hush as diners nudged one another and stared, aghast. Bob and Betty ignored the rude intrusion as the hostess showed them to their table, her eyes downcast, as she set their menus down. Bob carried a special chair for Susie that held her rigid body almost straight up for feedings. The busboy, an African American teenager, refused eye contact as he went about their table. He turned abruptly and left.

Andrew was beside himself with anger. He stared downward, his jaw clenching and unclenching. Bob was helping Betty get Susie into her special high chair.

There were more stares.

"Andrew, Honey, please stop it. We're at the dinner table," whispered Betty.

Angrily, Andrew stood and forcefully shoved his chair back, gaining even more unwanted attention as he stomped off to the men's room.

Bob stood, leaned over to Betty, and said, "Hold the fort down. We'll be right back."

In the men's room, Andrew stood with his forehead resting on the cold tiled wall with his hands clenched. Tears streamed down his face. Bob quietly entered. "What's this all about, Son?" asked Bob.

"Billy killed my dog!"

"I'm so sorry, Andrew. Maybe it was just an unfortunate accident," comforted Bob.

"No! It wasn't! There's a lock on the gate. Someone had to unlock it. Billy did that and he let Queenie out to get killed!" Andrew cried. "I hate Billy!"

Bob chose his words carefully. "I understand you're upset, son. What happened to Queenie was terrible. But you mustn't hate Billy. Instead, you must pray for him. Your mother and I are doing what we can for him. I haven't told your mother yet, but I don't think he's going to be with us much longer."

Andrew didn't respond.

"Son, God loves Billy too, and we must trust Him with his future. The LORD will work it out."

"I'm joining the navy," announced Andrew defiantly.

"What?" Bob was surprised. "Where did that come from? You're too young, Andrew."

Andrew replied, "I'm almost seventeen."

Bob snapped. "That's right, you are. And you have a lot of choices for your future in front of you. You needn't make any decisions now. You had better not say that to your mother. This will upset her even more."

"I'm not too young to join. I can join if you and Mom sign the papers. Naval recruiters came to our school last week. They're going to come to the house and talk to us about it."

Bob was stunned. "We'll talk about this when we get home. Now let's get back to the table. Not a word of this conversation to your mother."

***

When the family arrived back home, there was no time for Andrew and Bob to talk. Marion was sitting on the family room couch, a forlorn look on her face. Andrew went directly to his room and slammed the door hard.

Marion was the first to speak. "I hope you had a nice dinner."

Silence.

Marion continued, "I will call you tomorrow after I speak with social services first thing in the morning. We'll have time to talk then. In the meantime, I hope you have a quiet rest of your evening."

Betty didn't respond.

"I'll show you out, Marion," offered Bob.

"Thank you," she replied.

That evening in the privacy of their bedroom, Bob and Betty were both exhausted. More tears came when they hugged each other. Through a shaky, emotional voice, Betty said, "I don't understand what has happened to Billy. What did we do?"

"Honey," Bob assured her, "we didn't do anything. We gave an abandoned child a loving home rooted in the love of our LORD. Our job is to plant the seeds, but the outcome to our children's lives are up to them and their own choices to either live God's way or their own ways. We don't have the ability to control Billy's behavior, and frankly, I don't think he does either. Right now, all we can do is pray and put this situation into the hands of the LORD. His ways are not ours, and we need to trust in Him for the answer."

Return to Sender

The next morning was filled with tension. Neither Andrew nor Billy showed up for breakfast. Betty was clearing dishes when the phone rang. Bob answered it.

"Yes, Marion, of course. We will be there." Bob placed the phone back in its cradle. He said quietly, "Marion would like to meet us in Judge Lubarsky's office at ten this morning. She wants us to bring Billy."

Betty was alarmed. Bob continued, "Andrew can watch the children." Bob left the kitchen. "Andrew, can you come to the family room for a moment?" His voice trailed off.

***

In one hour, Bob, Betty, and Billy were in Judge Lubarsky's office with Marion Brown. Marion had a thick file in her hands and a somber look on her face. After the formalities, the session began.

Marion handed the file to Judge Lubarsky who took nearly a quarter of an hour going through it. The room was silent. Betty nervously clung to Bob's arm, worried and scared. In the meantime, Billy started kicking Bob's chair and wouldn't stop after several reprimands. Then he got quiet. Something else caught his attention.

Suddenly, he jumped out of his chair and lunged toward the judge's desk. Billy grabbed the letter opener and menacingly approached the judge with it. Judge Lubarsky grabbed the phone.

"Miss Jenkins, get Officer Jones in here at once," he barked.

Officer Jones was in the judges' chambers in seconds, and immediately, he was wrestling the letter opener out of Billy's hand. Billy smirked as the officer led him out of the office. Betty started to protest, but Bob put a protective hand over hers.

Judge Lubarsky closed the file, removed his glasses, and leaned forward. "Billy has been diagnosed with severe reactive attachment disorder (RAD) with a mounting evidence of psychosis, and from the reports that his social worker has written, his condition is only worsening. These are both dangerous conditions that will only worsen in time. For your safety and the safety of your family, I have no other choice than to order that he be removed from your home immediately."

Betty gasped. Bob grabbed her hand.

Marion intervened. "Bob, Betty, you have done so much for Billy. You absolutely cannot blame yourselves for any of this. These are psychiatric disorders that need full-time treatment and supervision. He is a danger to your family, and he cannot be allowed to stay with you any longer."

"But what will happen to him?" Betty cried.

Judge Lubarsky said firmly but quietly, "I have made arrangements for Billy to be placed in a boys home in another state where he will be constantly supervised and get the psychiatric care he needs."

Judge Lubarsky paused as he read something in Billy's file. He let out a sigh and shook his head. "I see here that Billy's biological mother was a prostitute who was stabbed to death by her client in front of him when he was three years old, one year before he came to you. This is an unbelievable trauma this boy has suffered. Looking back, I'm not sure why he was even placed up for adoption as for sure he was bound to have a severe psychiatric disorder of some sort."

Betty was aghast. Bob asked, "Will we be allowed to visit him at least?"

"No, I'm very sorry. It won't do any of you any good. It is best that you sever all ties with him." The judge was quiet for a moment. "Mr. and Mrs. Smith, I am very aware of your amazing family and the work you do with these children. I can only assure you that you did everything possible for Billy. You can have peace in your family now without having all of these disruptions. I wish you only the best."

"Can we at least say goodbye to him?" requested Betty.

"Yes, of course, you can. This case is now closed," replied Judge Lubarsky.

Betty, Bob, and Marion left quietly.

***

Officer Jones stepped aside and opened the door to the small room where Billy sat on a chair, kicking his legs. He didn't look up when his parents entered. Betty was shaking as she leaned over to give her first adopted son a hug. He reacted by nearly kicking her in the shins. Bob pulled her away as Billy sat on the chair and let out a laugh that was almost a cackle. He stared straight ahead, not making any effort to have eye contact with either of them. A warm goodbye was useless, and Bob understood that as he led his wife out of the room.

A Quieted Family

As soon as Bob and Betty returned home, they couldn't help but notice the immediate calm that came over the family. Still, what lingered was their heartbreak over the loss of their child and the terrible sense of failure that they had somehow let Billy down. Not since the passing of Joseph had they experience such a sense of devastation. This episode was especially terrible for Andrew who had so badly wanted a sibling. Now Andrew had lost his beloved dog Queen because of the behavior of his first adopted brother, and he was inconsolable. There was an anger brewing inside of Andrew neither of them had seen before, and it was terribly unsettling. Unspoken between them, if the other children were not already adopted, they would not have dared to adopt again. There was no way of ever knowing how their earlier traumas were to affect them in the years to come no matter how much love an adoptive parent was willing to give. What sustained them in these terrible, sad hours was that their other children, for now, continued to bless them.

Andrew's reaction was to withdraw from his family. Betty and Bob decided to let him alone and allow him to grieve in private because they knew how much he had loved Queenie. Even though Billy was gone, they both understood that Andrew had to have time to heal. Andrew was almost seventeen, and his immediate concern was what he was going to do once he got out of high school. They had always believed that becoming a chiropractor was what he wanted. There had even been an opportunity for him to stay with a family friend in Illinois where he could go to school. "I can't bear the thought of Andrew moving away, especially now," Betty had mentioned. But Andrew had done what was expected of him and had stayed with their family friend, but it had not worked out. Now everything about Andrew's future was up in the air.

The Hunt for Andrew Jerome Smith

The doorbell rang. Bob excused himself and went to answer it. In the porch light, he could see two men in naval uniforms.

"Who's at the door, Honey?" called Betty.

Bob was standing in the doorway staring at the two naval officers on the porch when his wife joined him.

The taller one spoke first, "Mr. and Mrs. Smith? I'd like to introduce myself. I am Petty Officer Mike O'Brien, and this is Petty Officer William Lucas. Your son, Andrew, has expressed interest in joining the navy, and we're here to sit down and talk with all of you about it." With all the drama with Billy, Bob had completely forgotten to mention the conversation he had had with Andrew in the men's room in the restaurant to Betty.

"The navy!" Betty blurted out. "Andrew wants to join the navy? He most certainly—"

"Honey, why don't you get the men settled in the dining room, and I'll go get Andrew," said Bob as he took Betty by her elbow. He had to shove her gently to get her to move.

Gathered around the dining room table, Andrew eagerly soaked up every word said. Bob looked quietly at the brochures of beautiful seas and sandy seashores and application forms with a look of serious uncertainty on his face. Betty glared unmercifully at the two recruiters. She didn't say a word. She began to blank out.

Tears of a Mother

"Vietnam," said Recruiter Lucas, "is not something to worry about. After all, it has never been officially declared a war."

"Will I travel overseas?" Andrew asked excitedly.

Recruiter O'Brien looked directly at Betty. "You give your son to us, and we'll return him to you a man."

Betty glared daggers. O'Brien's eyes were rimmed in red. His pupils dilated, then turned into vertical slits, gold slits, like a cat. His skin was gray; his mouth was moving. "You give your son to us—"

"And we'll return him to you a man," continued Lucas. He smiled. In place of teeth were long, long pointed fangs. They dripped with blood. His hot, sour, stinking breath blew in Betty's face.

She recoiled, gagging.

"Sign the papers. He's underage. He's ours now." Recruiter O'Brien shoved the papers toward Bob who didn't move.

Betty' and Bob's lips were moving, but no sounds came out. They were asking questions and making comments, all unheard. Betty started yelling, "We won't sign the papers! You can't take our son!"

Betty was not heard.

The recruiters stood and smiled through their cat eyes and blood-dripping fangs. "If you won't sign the papers, we'll just have to take him."

Andrew stood excitedly, at attention, and saluted, ignoring his frantic parents.

Recruiter Lucas offered his hand to Bob; only his fingers were claws. Bob recoiled. He grabbed Betty by her collar and pulled her back with him.

Betty let out a terrifying scream. She was still screaming, unheard, as the two recruiters surrounded Andrew and lifted him up. The trio ascended into oblivion. Andrew was gone!

Goodbye, Andrew

For the next two years, Bob and Betty could think of little else but their son leaving them to join the navy, and they dreaded the inevitable. Their son had never gotten over his pain and anger at losing his beloved dog Queenie, and all he wanted from that point on was get away from his painful memories as quickly as he could. Although neither Bob nor Betty could ever admit it, Andrew had turned on them. The navy would take him far, far away, and that's what he wanted. Now that he was eighteen, he was more determined than ever to join the navy regardless of his parents painful, pleading protestations. Unspoken, at least to Andrew, was their deep concern about Vietnam even though, at that point, nothing official was happening yet. And now, they were driving him to Chicago O'Hare airport to send him off into the unknown. Saying goodbye to Andrew was almost more than either of them could bear.

Andrew could barely keep himself contained; his excitement was so great, but at least, he still had some sensitivity to somewhat control himself around his parents in those final moments. But his mind was made up. He graduated high school and even attended a chiropractor school while he waited for his orders. To his friends, he was a hero for making such a bold move against his parents, wishes to serve his country and leave the comforts of home.

The car approached the sign for the passenger drop-off. "Hey, Dad, just pull up and let me off here."

Bob was angered, then quietly said, "No, Son, we are going inside together and seeing you off as a family." As always, all the children were in the car, most of them having no real understanding of the enormity of the situation. For Andrew, he was finally on his way to freedom. The last thing he wanted was an emotional scene in the airport gate area, but he would endure it because the next step would be to get on the plane so he could fly away to freedom. He leaned back and didn't say a word as Bob searched for a parking space.

The Final Countdown

The arrival at the gate was agony for Bob and Betty. Some of the children were excited about being inside the airport that was a bit of a nice diversion for their parents. A few passengers graciously stood with the usual nudges and stares, offering their seats that Bob and Betty thankfully accepted. Andrew was lost in thought. About all Betty could come up with to say was "Don't forget to write." Andrew promised to write, but his attention was more focused on the boarding gate than his mother. Time passed uncomfortably slow. Finally, the flight was called. Andrew issued his last hugs before excitedly joining the line to board the plane. Betty tried to bite back her tears, an unsuccessful endeavor. Late that evening, Bob and Betty knelt beside their bed. Bob prayed out loud from one of his favorite verses, Proverbs 3:5: "Trust in the Lord with all your heart and lean not on thy own understanding."

Bob turned to his grieving wife. "Honey, the LORD in His wisdom has given each one of us the freedom of choice, and Andrew has made his. We don't know what the consequences of his choices will be, but the LORD does. No matter what the outcome may be, we have to trust that the LORD's hand is in all things. All we can do now is keep Andrew in prayer and know that the LORD is in charge. Someday, we will understand."

Chapter 7

God's Many Miracles
1966–1974

Several Months Later

Less than a year had passed since Andrew joined the navy when Bob and Betty received a call from an adoption agency. Caucasian paternal twins, Rob and Rebecca (Becky), were five months old, and both were born with severely malformed cleft palates and suffered from projectile vomiting that was so forceful it covered the ceiling, walls, and anyone and anything else within vomiting distance. Their deformities were so severe Bob made the comment, "You can see the back of their throats from five feet away." The twins were scary thin from a lack of nourishment. The first thing on the Smiths' agenda was to keep them nourished and everything and everyone else clean, a seemingly hourly challenge. Thankfully, it wasn't long before the twins were able to undergo surgeries to close their palates.

Not long after, their newborn son James arrived. Of African American descent, his birth mother was an alcoholic, heroin-and-meth-addicted prostitute. Immediately at birth, he went through withdrawal, an indescribable, inhumane start to life. A beautiful boy, his life was to be filled with addictive cravings, emotional disturbances, and an inability to eat any foods that were processed or contained food dyes. Through no fault of his own, his emotions, psyche, and body couldn't deal with the cruelty of his mother's choices she inflicted upon him during her pregnancy. Relationships were difficult at best, and uncontrollable outbursts were frequent.

Still, Bob and Betty were very proud of James and loved him very much. They couldn't wait to show off their new son, so they attended a gathering of parents like themselves at a picnic. It was there they became aware of a baby boy who had the same background as James did. His name was Christopher, and he was biracial. Both his parents were alcoholics, and during his mother's pregnancy, she drank heavily. As a result, Christopher was born with fetal alcohol syndrome and cirrhosis of the liver. The foster home that cared for him was forced to close its doors due to neglect.

In no time at all, Bob, Betty, and James were introduced to Christopher, and they fell in love with him immediately. He was as strikingly handsome as James was. Through a two-way mirror in the counselor's office, they were able to watch as James and Christopher were brought together. They took an immediate liking to each other, and in that moment, their great affection and trust toward each other would prove to be lifelong. Bob and Betty nearly melted when they heard James say to Christopher, "You're my birthday present!" Within two months, Christopher was officially a member of their family and, most importantly, James's new brother. From that point on, the two boys were inseparable.

The Wonderful, Gracious Dr. Poitier

Early on when their children first began to arrive, Betty was led through a friend's referral to Dr. Poitier, a family physician. In her eyes, he was a godsend.

Dr. Poitier himself had a harelip, which is probably why he took such a special interest in every one of the Smiths' children. He was thorough, kind, compassionate, and encouraging.

"Well, who is this big handsome boy?" he said to a big, proud, and smiling Peter. "A little bird told me you're about to start kindergarten." He turned to Betty. "Isn't it amazing how healthy he is now? There's not even a trace of rickets, and he's growing up so fast. Look at his beautiful head of hair."

All Betty could do was smile. "Yes, he's very excited. We all are."

Next was Edwin. "You're growing up into a fine young man, Edwin. How are you?"

Edwin hung his head and remained silent.

Betty mentioned that Edwin was still in pain and emotionally unresponsive. "I'm worried about the bone chips.

He's in constant pain, but he never complains. All I have to do is look at him, and I see the pain in his face."

"I'll see what I can do for him today to help his pain. I'll prescribe a different medication, and we'll monitor him to see how he does. Let's watch and see if hopefully he will brighten up a bit."

Susie gurgled happily in her stroller. Dr. Poitier lifted the removable part of the stroller and put her on the exam table. He took his finger and moved it in front of her eyes. She tracked his finger from side to side, from farther away to up close. With a satisfied smile, he got out his stethoscope. Again, he smiled. He put the stethoscope down and turned toward Betty.

"The immediate great care you have given all of these children has saved them from what would have happened to these children if God hadn't sent them to you. Susie's surgeries to save her eyesight and to correct her congenital heart condition have given her a life with hope. There's been a breakthrough in treating cerebral palsy, and I'll see to it that she gets it. Edwin's trauma is being overcome with the love you and Mr. Smith give to him. Look at Peter, how healthy and big he is, and Christopher too. He is thriving in your home. Isn't God's timing perfect?" Betty choked back tears and nodded in agreement. "They're all miracles, each and every one of them." As an afterthought, he added, "I wonder how many more miracles God is going to send to you and Mr. Smith."

"We'll take all the miracles He sends us." Betty laughed.

A Small Taste of What Is Yet to Come

Betty was so proud of Peter who stood before her, barely five years old, all dressed and ready for his first day of kindergarten. She could tell he was nervous though. He fidgeted with his lunch pail while shifting from side to side with a look of uncertainty on his face.

Bob was traveling on that day, and Betty was alone, so Peter got to ride in the front seat with her on the way to school while the other younger children rode in the back seat. Edwin had gotten a ride to school with another mother and classmate for this special morning.

Betty never noticed that Peter's class was filled with all Caucasian children. She didn't really notice that those children had all stopped what they were doing, and they were staring at her dark-skinned son. She was focused on Peter alone, and choking back tears, she hugged him goodbye.

When Betty arrived after school to pick up her son, she noticed that Peter was very tense. His head hung, and he seemed closed off. This was not the happy little boy she was expecting to see.

As soon as Betty got Peter settled inside the car, he began to sob.

"Didn't you have a nice day, Sweetheart? What's wrong?" Betty asked anxiously.

"I'm your son. I'm not an Eskimo," he gulped. The teacher, in all her kindness, was trying to explain Peter's dark skin and almond-shaped eyes to the other students. Betty was furious and heartsick, but instead of confronting the teacher, she chose to stay calm for her son and drive him home.

"If Bob had been with me that day, something would have been said to the teacher," recalls Betty sadly. "But he wasn't, and all I wanted to do was comfort my son and get him back home. Looking back, I so much wish I had."

This was just the beginning for Peter who oftentimes felt himself shunned or pointed out because he was different to them. A neighbor had called him a "lazy Chicano," which caused him great upset. Angry, he started to act out, which became more pronounced in his later years.

Often, Peter found himself in trouble with the law, which infuriated him even more toward society and others around him. This same type of harassment was pointed at all the children, and many of them followed the same downward road. Peter was the first of their children to follow this path but certainly not the last, which caused Bob and Betty many sleepless nights. This ugly road to reality caused a great deal of harm to all of them. In later years though, Peter thankfully was able to turn his life around. Fortunately, through steady and loving guidance, discipline, and relentless prayer, Peter eventually became the loving young man he was intended to be.

The reality was several of their children did, or were going to, struggle with anger, and not all of them would be able to fully recover. Bob and Betty could only protect them to a certain point, and after that, they would have to stand on their own two feet. Every evening before going to bed, Bob and Betty were on their knees praying the same prayer they taught their children, 1 John 4:4: "You are from God, little children, and have overcome them; because greater is He who is in you is greater than he who is in the world."

Overcomers

When Susie was around twelve, she accomplished something that amazed the entire family. Close friends of the family were getting married. The couple asked that the children of their friends precede the bride down the aisle releasing balloons. As a gift to the bride and groom, Susie decided she wanted to walk down the aisle of the church unaided by her crutches. For weeks preceding the wedding, Betty took her to the church to practice alone with the organist. At that time of day, the sun shone through the stained-glass windows, its brilliant, radiant, dancing colors glimmering on Susie as she struggled, lurched, fell, and picked herself up again as she struggled to walk unaided down the aisle without any complaint. No one else was there to witness this miracle of determination except for her and the organist. Betty knelt, fervently praying one of her favorite scriptures she often prayed for each of her children, 1 John 4:4: "You are from God, little children, and have overcome them; because greater is He who is in you than he who is in the world." She watched Susie overcome, one step at a time, in complete awe of this miraculous sight.

On the wedding day, Susie achieved her dream of walking down the aisle unaided with the entire family and numerous friends in attendance. This was the beginning for Susie to walk unaided.

Around this time, Peter's suffering and his accompanying angry behavior landed him in constant trouble with the law. This was the ongoing terrible personal battle of prejudice and rejection. Inevitably, his anger and humiliation finally took its toll, and he turned on society and ended up in the courts. After much grief and heartbreak, Peter was eventually placed in White's Institute that was a boarding school for Indian children who needed supervision and an education.

"The owners were beautiful Quaker people who dearly loved him," Betty remembers. Through their support and guidance, Peter began to turn his life around. He not only graduated, he was asked to work there as the house supervisor.

In Heartbreak We Trust

For Bob and Betty, their overwhelming concern for Andrew was different. Not only was he Betty's first and only biological child and Bob's beloved first adopted son, he was now in harm's way. Onboard a hospital ship, he was seeing indescribable horrors as he tended to the wounded of Vietnam. Although his letters home were increasingly infrequent, Bob and Betty received each one with great trepidation. Thank God, he was still alive, but the horrors inflicted upon him and the change she could detect in his tone was often as painful as losing him to death, if not worse. Their son was in a living nightmare, and there was nothing they could do but pray for him.

The real trouble was detectable when Andrew worked as a photojournalist during the conflict. There he saw the real atrocities in action, not just their aftermath. It was during this time that his letters were nearly at a standstill. They could read how destroyed and despondent he was becoming. He no longer relayed events to her. In its place was anger. One comment set them both back terribly. "Mom, stop telling the children that the world is a beautiful place because this world is a living hell."

As Betty later began to suspect, Andrew had become involved in drugs. Gone was their once-sweet, loving boy. In his place was a young man filled with rage, bitterness, and despair. It began with him smoking hashish that in time led him to drugs that were far more dangerous. Helpless, all they could do was pray for their beloved son. Their worry for him never went away.

While waiting for Andrew's leave time, Bob and Betty were filled with great fear and concern. Anxious to see their son, they had no idea what to expect. The tone of his letters left little doubt that he was in terrible psychological and emotional turmoil. They were not prepared for his wild-eyed look and lashing out at everyone in sight. His behavior was so abusive there was little choice but to get him out of the house in order to protect their children. It was almost a relief when Andrew left to go back to Vietnam. Their first son was lost to them in a way they had never experienced; even the finality of death paled by comparison. They watched helplessly as their once-loving and considerate son turned into someone they no longer knew or could relate to. He endured experiences no human being could be expected to endure, and for him, there was no way out but through the temporary relief of mind-altering drugs that would later bring on their own ruinous consequences. They knew they had lost their son, but not to death. They lost him to a living hell, and it was a pain that was incomprehensibly excruciating. Andrew would be coming home for good soon, and they had no idea what to expect. Not for one day did Bob and Betty fail to pray for him. They had no choice but to trust the outcome to Jesus.

A Lost Soul

After Andrew's final return in 1974, Bob and Betty had to face the fact that he was destroyed. They did what they could by consulting doctors, pastors, and even to Vietnam veteran support groups, but to no avail. They did learn that their son was suffering from what is now known as post traumatic stress disorder (PTSD), but in those days, very little was known about it; therefore, little to nothing could be done for him. Andrew was drug and alcohol addicted. One day, Andrew left their home in a fit of anger and temper. Frankly, they were relieved, as his behavior had taken a terrible toll on all of them. Going a few months without communication had not been necessarily unusual, but when one year turned into two years, then even more years, they both became frightened for their son. They were so distressed Bob hired a private investigator that was able to trace him to Sacramento, California, but there the road came to an abrupt stop. In time, they both had to accept that their beloved Andrew was gone without any trace. Regardless, their grief was acute, and their hearts were absolutely shattered. It was the "not knowing" that crushed them. It was worse than death because at least, with death, there is closure; you get to say goodbye and bury someone. Day in and day out, they carried the sadness and heartache of uncertainty with them no matter what else was going on in their busy lives, and it was palpable.

"After Vietnam, Andrew was never the same. His disappearance nearly destroyed us," a heartbroken Betty whispered. "There are no lessons in life that teach you how to cope with that kind of heartbreak."

What Bob and Betty never expected was that they would lose their son Andrew forever.

It would be decades past Bob's death when Betty finally learned the terrible fate of her firstborn son.

Book 2

For I know the plans I have for you, plans to prosper you and not to harm you, plans to give you hope and a future.

—Jeremiah 29:11

Baby Hugh Dermott O'Connor

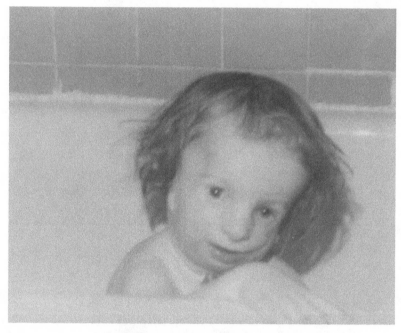

Soon-to-be Francis Joel Smith

Chapter 1

Hugh Dermott O'Connor
1977–1983

Start children off on the way they should go,
and even when they are old they will not turn from it.
— Proverbs 22:6

All of our kids were in the same boat. We were
a put-together family, and they knew it. They all
knew exactly from where they had come from.
— Betty Smith

***

The Smith Family (Late 1977)

"Betty, I am going to kick you in the shins if you don't stop it!"

Those were very stern hiss words from Betty Smith's dear friend Linda Matz, who had accompanied her to a convention for social workers in Indianapolis, Indiana. Already, Bob and Betty Smith were the adoptive parents of nine children of various races and levels of special needs. The Smiths—who now raised their brood in New Haven, a suburb of Fort Wayne, Indiana—were sought-after adoptive parent role models and speakers. Betty spoke that day to social workers from various adoption agencies about adopting children with challenges and special needs.

"There were so many children with challenges who needed homes, and families were afraid to take them, so they were not being placed," Betty said. "I recall saying, 'If you expect more from a child, you are going to get more.' I never talked about myself. I told them what would happen if they took a special needs child and gave them a chance."

Betty had barely finished her last words when Pat Vespers from Child Welfare Services rushed up to the podium and said, "Because of your speech, I have found a home for this very special child."

Betty was very excited over this news. She replied, "Who?"

"You!" replied Pat.

Linda came unglued. It was no secret she felt the Smiths had too many children as it was. She was furious!

Yet Betty was already very well aware who this "very special child" was, and *she* was excited! "There was a catalog we had from the adoption agency that Bob and I belonged to that kept up with children with special needs who were up for adoption. Every month, we were sent a new photograph of these children, so each month, I replaced the old photograph of Hugh with the new one. All of our children watched as he grew and grew. The adoption group we belonged to also adopted biracial children with special needs. Four of our nine children were biracial."

As soon as Betty returned late that evening, she couldn't wait to tell Bob what had transpired. But he insisted that the children make the decision, not themselves. That night, they knelt beside their bed and prayed for each child by name as they always did. This time, they asked the LORD if it was His will that Hugh become a part of their family.

"There were seven other children in our house who all wanted attention," reminds Betty. "Bob traveled a lot, so I was left alone with all of our children quite a bit. All of our kids were in the same boat. We were a put-together family, and they knew it. They all knew exactly from where they had come from.

"The next evening, we all sat at around the large round coffee table with its shortened legs for our nightly reading of *Our Daily Bread* before dinner. Not one of the children asked me about the conference. Finally, Bob said, 'Nobody has asked your mother about her speaking engagement yesterday.'

"'Oh, yeah, Mom, how did it go?'

"That's when I told them about Hugh. Bob was very gung ho about taking the 'little guy', but I never thought for a moment the kids would go for it—but they did. We didn't yet know the entire story about Hugh. Actually, I was very apprehensive."

Right then and there, the children unanimously voted Hugh into their family.

The Road to Reality

The next day, Betty contacted Pat Vespers and told her the family was ready to start the steps of bringing Hugh into the Smith family, a process that was bound to be a lengthy one. Almost immediately, Bob and Betty were scheduled to meet Hugh at the Child Welfare Social Services Division in Indianapolis.

"I remember Bob and I were very nervous while sitting in the waiting room," reminisced Betty. "Then Hugh was brought in. He just stared at us for the longest time; then he started to twirl, round and round. He didn't stop!"

After the initial meeting, Bob and Betty were more smitten with Hugh than ever. Betty committed to making as many trips into Indianapolis to Mrs. Collins's home as needed in order to learn Hugh's complex care routine. Her very good friend, Lee Durland, a psychiatric nurse, planned to always go with her.

Mrs. Collins and her two daughters lived in a terribly rundown, rough section of Indianapolis. It simply was not an area that two women should be driving around in, especially not alone. The dilapidated house had an unkempt lawn, peeling paint, and torn curtains. The neighborhood literally came to a stop as tough-looking kids and neighbors began peeking through their curtains watching with blank faces as Betty and Lee parked the car and nervously made their way up the pathway to the front door. Upon ringing the doorbell, a dark-skinned young woman pulled back the frayed curtain and looked them in the eye before letting the curtain go and answered the door.

Betty and Lee were greeted by one of the most loving, brightest, shining grins they had ever witnessed. The young woman graciously invited them in. One step inside, they noticed that the wood floor was badly splintered, and the walls were in dire need of paint. They were led to a closed, locked door. She unlocked the door, and inside a crib was Hugh who was standing and staring at his visitors.

Hugh was crib bound, not out of meanness but for his safety. The splintered floor was dangerous, but more threatening to him were a couple of other children Mrs. Collins and her daughters fostered. His door was kept locked.

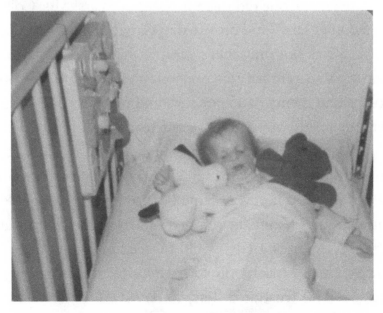

A safe haven for Hugh

"How well do I remember the trips made to Mrs. Collins's home, a home full of love as she and her daughters cared for Hugh and other foster children before they were adopted," remembers Lee.

"When I first met Hugh, he was very thin, large eyes, no ears, no chin with a large tongue hanging out. He didn't cry or smile. He looked like a shrunken adult in the body of a one-year-old, and he was two and a half years old!"

The women watched with awe as Mrs. Collins painstakingly fed Hugh through gavage tubing with a syringe while she also suctioned the tracheostomy to make sure it was always clean and cleared. "With every feeding, the clean tubing had to be inserted through the nostril, past the cleft palate and down the esophagus, and after the feeding, it had to be removed. She did this for over two years! Mrs. Collins was another saint God provided to care for Hugh," said Lee.

Lee was not only there for moral support but also to learn how to care for this precious young boy. While Mrs. Collins had plenty of experience and made it appear fairly easy, the reality was it was a very frustrating learning curve. There was so much more to learn beyond the obvious. The gavage tube itself was a source of constant frustration to both women, as it never seemed to go where it was guided, but instead, it habitually popped out from the cleft palate. After several tries, Betty would succeed in getting the tube down to his stomach only to have his feedings come right back up! This frustrated Betty to tears.

"Just be thankful he has no ears," joked Lee. "Otherwise, the tube would come out there too!"

There were times when Betty got so nervous and frustrated she wanted to quit. But as they got better at it, surprisingly, Hugh thrived on the attention and was unusually patient during their practice sessions.

"One time, I was particularly nervous. I had my car keys in my hand, and I was jiggling them because I wanted to go. Hugh was fixated on them. He grabbed them! I said, 'No!' I grabbed them back. Mrs. Collins came over and told me I couldn't say no to Hugh. But I had to. I needed the car keys to go home. So I said no, and that was that. I was ready to back out the door and leave."

This is Francis's first memory in his life.

"I remember the first thing that attracted me to my new mom was her set of keys attached to a humongous blue round plastic key tag. To me, it was a fascinating new toy, and I wanted it immediately! I used the same old trick that had worked with Mrs. Collins; I threw a whopping temper tantrum when Mom refused to just hand them over to me. Mrs. Collins advised Mom that I was a ferocious tantrum thrower and that she should hand over her keys, or I would really launch into a strong tantrum. Surprisingly, Mom held her ground and stood up to me; she needed those keys to get home! I would soon find out that unlike Mrs. Collins, Mom was not an easy person to control with my temper."

Eventually, Mrs. Collins came to accept that Hugh was going to a very loving home. As difficult as it was to part ways with her young boy, it was agreed that whenever the Smiths had to visit Riley Hospital, Mrs. Collins would become a part of the trip.

Francis remembers fondly, "My parents and I kept her updated on my life, and once, I sent her a tape of one of my piano recitals. Often, we would visit with her and her daughters for an hour or more. Over the years, Mrs. Collins, Mom, and I maintained a very close friendship. The last time I visited her was in 1990, shortly before she died at a ripe old age. I still have the stuffed mouse she and her daughters gave me at the last visit. I miss her today, but I know for sure she is in the loving arms of her Maker, where I will someday meet her again."

"The last trip I accompanied Betty to Mrs. Collins's home was to pick up Hugh to take him to the Smith home as their legal child," Lee said. "It was getting late, and as we drove out of Indianapolis and got on the circumferential highway, we missed the turn off to Fort Wayne twice, having circled Indianapolis twice before we realized what we had done. I guess our excuse was that it was dark, and we were talking excitedly about Hugh, about what can be done medically and surgically about his handicaps, and he was as quiet as a mouse, sitting in the back seat, snuggled tightly in the child's car seat.

"Love means different things to different people, but when I saw the Smith family every Sunday walk up the aisle of our church in Fort Wayne with their multiple adopted children, it was a beautiful sight to behold," claims Lee. "Bob and Betty Smith knew and practiced what love was all about. Oh, they could've adopted two or three and would've had more time and money to take cruises and expensive vacations, but they chose to give their all to raising these special needs children. Now, adopting ten was extraordinary enough, but their hearts had been enlarged by their giving and giving of themselves to raising theirs to the point they found room for not just one more—Hugh AKA Francis—but eventually his younger sister, Ruth, as well. I believe he and Ruth were their most special ones because they were the most seriously handicapped.

"What a witness the Smith family is to agape love."

A Forever Family—New Haven, Indiana

Our children shaped everything we became.
It was they who turned our home into a Forever Home.
—Betty Smith

Prior to Hugh's arrival to the Smith household, Bob and Betty paid the local fire station a visit. They told them about a very unique little boy who had very special challenges who was coming to live with them. Their new son had problems that could not wait out being snowed in. "We needed a lot of special foods and supplies to care for him, so snow could possibly present a real problem for us. They agreed to help us out if we got snowed in. And they did!" That very winter, the Smiths got snowed in, and the firemen arrived on snowmobiles carrying the supplies that were needed.

Amazingly, the transition from Mrs. Collins's home into the hectic family lifestyle of the Smith household appeared not to faze Hugh in the slightest. Mrs. Collins had made the transition as easy as possible by allowing Betty and Francis to form a very strong bond before the move was made.

"The family I joined was a large one," remembers Francis. "The home in New Haven was buzzing with the activity of five other adopted children plus dogs and cats. The two eldest, Peter and Edwin, were grown by then and off on their own. All of my siblings were adopted from various backgrounds and came into the family with their own unique challenges, some physical and others not as visible. Mom and Dad had devoted their entire marriage to taking in all these children and caring for them; over the years since the sixties, children came one after the other or sometimes in twos. By the time I joined the family in 1978, our home was a virtual United Nations of children from all kinds of backgrounds."

Immediately, the entire household was enamored with Hugh, and he reveled in all their attention. Hugh didn't arrive at the Smith family home alone. He brought along all his baggage that his two and a half years of life required. His medical needs alone were daunting and ongoing. His tracheostomy tube required constant suctioning several times a day. The tiny silver trach tubes had to be changed, cleaned, sterilized, and polished, a never-ending job. He could never ever be left alone, not even for just a few minutes. When an emergency hit— like it often did—it would hit without warning. The most common emergency was a tube blockage caused by an unclean tube or, worse, food that was accidentally sucked into his lungs that would then cause respiratory distress. The Smiths became very adept at handling these emergencies without batting an eyelash.

"Peter and Edwin would drop over nearly every day to help with the gavage feedings and chores. I, or Peter, would hold him while the other would attempt to thread the tube through his nostril, down his esophagus and into his stomach. Then the solution was poured into a syringe barrel on the outside end of the tube in order for it to flow down by gravity into his stomach. More often than not, as soon as the solution hit his stomach, it would come right back up again and, all over, everything and everyone," recalled Betty. The solutions were so-called recipes sent over from Riley Hospital. Blended, liquefied carrots seemed to be the most-often vegetable of choice to the point where Francis began to turn a sickly orange color. Although he remains underweight to this day, those multiple feedings in his earlier years undoubtedly is what kept him alive.

"The rest of our children helped a great deal as they had all along with one another. Some would sit with Hugh and spin toys around and around. They all pitched in," continued Betty. "We didn't have many problems at all. We never had outside help; we had inside help. All of our children know exactly where they came from. Francis became our tenth adopted child."

For the love of family.

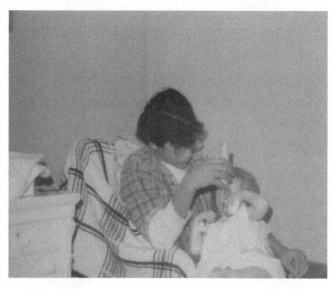

Peter feeding Francis through his gavage tube.

A New Beginning for Hugh

The first order of family business was getting their newest adopted child baptized. The Smiths were members of a local Catholic church at that time, the faith Bob had been reared in. It was his desire that the spiritual faith he cherished be the foundation upon which his marriage and growing family would thrive on. Their newest son arrived into the family as Hugh Dermott O'Connor, a name that had no meaning to the Smiths. The night before his baptism, Bob announced he wanted to change Hugh's name. Once again, the family gathered around the shortened round coffee table to discuss what their new son and brother would be called.

Observed Betty, "My husband loved St. Francis of Assisi and said that Francis reminded him of this saint. So that's how he became Francis." The others came up with Joel as his middle name.

"Bob asked their parish priest, Father Tom, if he would do the honors. The poor man was scared to death," remembered Betty. While the family was accustomed to Hugh's disturbing appearance, others were not. Human nature being what it is, most reacted to him by recoiling and turning away.

The next morning, in front of the statue of St. Francis of Assisi and the entire congregation, Hugh Dermott O'Connor was baptized with his new name, Francis Joel Smith.

Introducing Francis Joel Smith

Immediately after Francis's baptism, the most important "to do" was for Betty to take their new son to see Dr. Poitier. On that particular day, neither Rob or Edwin were able to sit with the other children, so this meant that she had to bring younger children with her, five in all, including Francis.

Visiting their beloved Dr. Poitier was usually not a problem. There had always been some reaction from other patients when Betty brought her children in, but this time, she found herself in the center of an extremely embarrassing situation. No sooner had they entered the waiting room than the door to the hall that led to the exam room was flung open. Without preamble, a new nurse stood in the doorway and ordered Betty to get into the exam room. "The appearances of your children are frightening the other children and their mothers. Please go directly to the exam room," she said sternly and loudly. Mortified, Betty did as she was told. The nurse just stood there, not offering any assistance as Betty struggled into the exam room.

Once inside, the new nurse continued with her rude tirade. "From now on when you have an appointment, you are not to settle in the waiting area. You are to go directly into the exam room." Betty was speechless. Before the nurse left, she told Betty the children had to be weighed. "I'll start with the baby."

Betty, furious, bit her tongue. When the nurse came back to get Francis, he was stark naked. Without bothering to cover him up, she placed him face down over her arm and strutted past the door to the waiting room that was still open. From where Betty sat, she could hear and see their reactions to her son.

"Francis looked like a plucked chicken," Betty gasped. "He was emaciated, pale, and had various tubes and that terrible headgear on him and that awful woman went past the open door so everyone could see him. I was horrified and furious! I told her in no uncertain terms that she was to cover him up before she ever did anything like that again."

Before Betty could recover from her tirade, Dr. Poitier entered the exam room. In spite of his own harelip, he was smiling ear to ear. He was just beaming. In that moment, Betty forgot her own anger and found herself smiling with him.

"I see you have met my new wife," he stated. Betty's jaw dropped to the floor. "We got married two months ago. It's wonderful being able to work with her."

Not knowing what to say, she clammed up and started talking about the children.

The incident quickly forgotten, Betty and Dr. Poitier discussed Francis's cleft palate, his hearing, and various other maladies while he admired all the other children. He cared so deeply about all of them, but she could tell he had formed his most special bond with Francis.

Upon leaving, Betty had to go through the waiting room. Just as the door closed behind her in the hallway, she clearly heard the new Mrs. Poitier who was standing in the waiting room say, "How many husbands has that woman had?"

Dr. Poitier was quickly divorced.

***

As the next few weeks and months passed by, no one really knew for sure if Francis was able to hear. Not only was he nonverbal, he didn't even cry. Mrs. Collins had conveyed to Betty she believed Francis was deaf. After all, solid skull bone covered both ear canals. She briefly attended a school for the deaf to learn new skills in order to help him in any way she could.

"Mrs. Collins gave us a book filled with practical information," remembers Betty, "but we still weren't sure."

What Francis lacked in communication skills, he made up for with his whopping temper tantrums he seemingly threw at will, especially and always when Betty was about to leave. His personality was that of a determined, desperate child who was trying to survive and deal with frustrations he had no real ability to communicate in a way any of them could understand.

"Some would sit with Franny, as his family now called him, and spin toys around and around. They all pitched in," continued Betty. "We didn't have many problems at all. We never had outside help; we had inside help. All of our children remember exactly where they came from."

Necessary surgeries and ongoing medical care were simply a part of life in the Smith household. When one child was in need of special medical care, the others sprang into action to share responsibilities and care for one another.

There had been a gap of nearly seven years since their last adopted child joined the household, and thankfully, their medical needs were stable. At birth, Francis faced immediate surgery to save his life. Now that he was three years old, it was necessary to begin the numerous required surgeries that would help him live a more normal life.

Love lifted me.

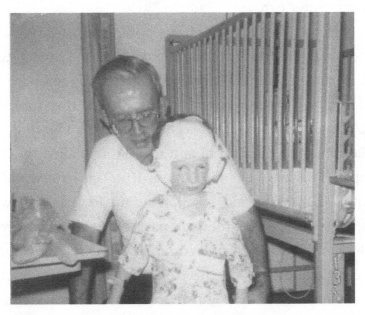

Bob with Francis in the hospital
after one of his surgeries.

Francis's multiple maladies aside, what concerned Bob and Betty the most was his hearing because their youngest child still could not speak.

Bob and Betty vowed to do anything and everything to help their newest child move forward in life, just as they had with all their children. An audiologist was consulted. Mrs. Collins had already gotten him a hearing aid, but it turned out that it wasn't the type he needed and had actually been useless. What Francis needed was some type of bone conduction hearing aid, a device that would pick up the sounds around Francis and send them to a vibrating earpiece strapped to his temple where the sound energy would be vibrated through the bone and into his inner ear.

"I remember my first bone conduction hearing aid," remembers Francis. "My audiologist led Mom and Dad to a headband-mounted hearing aid with a body-worn battery pack. It had a chrome body battery pack that took one AAA battery. A long cord connected it to a vibrating earpiece mounted on a headband to hold it against my right temple. This device finally opened me up to a world of sound. The hearing aid, by allowing me to hear somewhat properly for the first time ever, paved the way for my eventually learning to speak and communicate effectively during my early childhood. The hearing aid helped get me out of my autistic world—my autistic tendencies likely stemmed from my inability to hear. As I became able to hear with the aid, I began to emerge from my silent inner world and participate in the real world of sound and communication.

"It was hoped that the bone conduction hearing aid would be a temporary step because Mom and Dad wanted to eventually have my blocked ear canals opened," Francis continued. "They consulted with an ear surgeon at Riley Hospital to explore the possibility of reconstructing my ear canals. At age three, I was taken into the Riley Hospital operating room, where the doctor began to open one of my temples and explore my middle and inner ear structures to see how badly they were malformed. His hope was to go on during the same procedure to rebuild my ear canals. However, during the exploration of my ear, he found that it would be very risky to drill ear canals into my ears, as he was afraid the surgery would permanently damage my delicate inner ear structures. He had to close up the ear he was exploring and tell my parents that the procedure would be impossible and unnecessarily risk what little hearing I had. Thus, the bone-conduction hearing aid became a permanent part of my life to this day."

Another problem that needed attention was Francis's gaping cleft palate. Also at Riley Hospital and again at age three, Bob and Betty consulted with Dr. Stanley, one of the few plastic surgeons practicing there. At that time, the hospital had no craniofacial surgery team or program for dealing with the complicated needs of children like Francis who had severe craniofacial disorders. Dr. Stanley specialized in cleft palates, so he agreed to close his palate up the best he could. Francis went into surgery where the procedure to close the huge cleft in his palate began.

"When I came out, my palate was closed, except for a fistula, or tiny hole, that was unavoidably left between my hard and soft palates. This fistula would have to be closed several years later by yet another surgeon at another children's hospital," said Francis.

The repair of his cleft palate at that time though, along with the bone conduction hearing aid and Betty's diligent one-on-one work with him, were all contributors toward Francis's eventually learning to talk.

A rather surprising factor that was discovered after his cleft palate was closed was Francis actually had been able to "hear" all along—through his cleft palate! After his cleft palate was closed, he actually was completely deaf.

Ongoing Craniofacial Changes

Together, everyone pitched in to try and help Francis come out of his inner world. Slowly, his issues were addressed, one by one. Francis had to keep breathing through the tracheostomy until he was five years old. Aside from the immense full-time job keeping his trach in top working order, it also kept him from entering into society. Out in the brutal, hard, cold real world, he was kept out of preschool because teachers and children were afraid of his maladies and tubes. At last, after years of trying to convince his doctors it would be safe to do so, Dr. Singer—ear, nose, and throat doctor (ENT) at Riley Hospital—finally allowed the trach to be discontinued. However, Francis's gavage feeding was not.

In an effort to wean Francis off the gavage feedings, Betty started training him to take soft food and liquids by mouth with a baby spoon and sipper cup. The challenge was his severe large cleft palate and other deformities in his mouth. Betty never gave up. After a lengthy and determined effort, she was rewarded when her son was finally safely able to take food and liquid by mouth.

Next on the list was some badly needed dental work, difficult at best because of his ongoing craniofacial changes. This procedure was to be done in a Fort Wayne dental office while Francis was under nitrous oxide gas; then it was expected he would be taken home.

Partway through the oral procedure, Francis went into respiratory arrest, and he nearly died in the chair. Thankfully, the dentist's office immediately called 911. EMTs and fire-fighters revived him with his frightened mother praying in the room. After that experience, all his further dental work was done in the dental clinic at Riley Hospital.

Baidinger-Walter Funeral Home

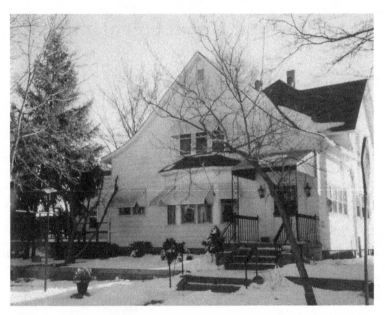

The Smith family's new home.

By wisdom a house is built, and by understanding
it is established; and by knowledge the rooms are
filled with all precious and pleasant riches.

—Proverbs 24:3–4

Chapter 2

A Funeral Home Full of Life
1979

The Breath of Life

Less than one year after Francis joined the Smiths, just short of the holidays, it was decided that a larger home was in order. In February 1979, Bob and Betty packed up their seven children and moved from their split-level home with green shutters in New Haven to a large white house in the nearby town of Garrett. Moving day coincided with a terrible blizzard that buried the entire Fort Wayne area under a thick white blanket of snow.

The Smiths' new home was distinctly unusual. Before they bought it, it had been the former Baidinger-Walter Funeral Home. For years, it sat on the market, empty, after their competitor, McKee Miles Funeral Home, bought them out. Garrett was much too small of a town to need two funeral homes. Even though the price steadily dropped, there were still no takers. No one wanted to live in a building where the dead lay in wait for their final resting place. When the realtor heard about the Smiths and how they were looking for a home for their seven children, she approached them, and not surprisingly, they accepted the low, low price of twenty-one thousand dollars—unheard of.

This was the perfect home for the large Smith family. The house had six bedrooms, all wood floors, french doors, and wainscoting all throughout. The front parlor had a large bay window and a huge gas fireplace. The kitchen was fairly small, but it had lots of cabinets with a very large dining room right off it. The rooms all had french doors, so it was easy for the children with mobility issues to move around. The home also had a large elevator for the caskets that was perfect for the children with wheelchairs or crutches. The embalming room was made into a huge shower and laundry room.

Remembers Betty, "When we first saw that room, it had huge hooks hanging from the ceiling. I was told that was where they hung the bodies! Oh! I made them take the hooks down right away! We also placed a large freezer in there. That worked out perfectly for our needs."

Francis has his own memories. "I remember the day we first entered the home; it was large, quiet, and empty. It was still decorated as a somber funeral home—with ivory paint and fancy formal wallpaper and heavy drapes all over, especially in the former front viewing room. Another room had a 'crossing over' bridge-over-a-river mural painted on one wall. There was still a platform lift in one of the two garages that was once used for bringing caskets and bodies into the back of the house from the garage. Also in the back of the house was the former embalming room with a basinlike linoleum floor with a drain in it. But the house had great potential for our large family. It had a dining room and kitchen, and we transformed the former casket selection room and chapels into living spaces with a parlor, playroom, and family room. We even had our own 'barbershop' in the back foyer. Dad would regularly line us boys up and cut our hair with his old barber tools."

Upstairs were five spacious bedrooms with each one painted a different color. Francis moved into the beige bedroom at the top of the stairs. "Our family transformed what had once been a home that dripped with the sorrow and finality of death to a lively, happy family home where each individual life was special and celebrated with joy. The first few years were spent fixing it up; my parents and siblings redecorated the main floor with brighter colors, covering up the dreary formal decor. The floors were repaired. We tore up old carpeting and varnished the pristine wood flooring that lay underneath. We insulated the house, making it warm in winter and cool in summer. Walls were repainted in brighter colors, and the dreary 'crossing-over' mural was painted over. A new roof eventually went on the house. One year, some of my older brothers helped build a wooden deck onto the front of the house for family cookouts and gatherings.

"We breathed life into our new home with all our activities. Around our large low round table, we sat and had our family time together as we watched TV, played games, and read our nightly readings of *Our Daily Bread* before dinner. Most of us learned to walk around that table. Our new playroom was roomy enough for our toys and games. It became our family recreational center where even some of my brothers played football games in the playroom!"

The World According to Francis

While focusing on Francis's obvious physical challenges, what crept up on the family were the complex emotional aspects of his personality that were deeply hidden but were becoming more and more apparent as time passed. Bob and Betty were completely frustrated because if they couldn't identify it, how could they deal with it?

"Francis was unable to express emotions. He was flat, therefore emotionally nonresponsive. For hours at a time, he would hold his fingers up to his face, wiggling and studying them," recalled Betty. "It was all very sad. Francis wanted so badly to make friends. He would sit in the backyard and make friends with rocks. He would 'talk' to them in his own special little language. He has such a loving demeanor. Everyone wanted to help him. He never asked for anything. He never did anything wrong. He was never malicious. He was never depressed. He adored all the attention he got from our family. Most of all, he knew he was loved.

"At his age of three years old, normal children are running around, playing games and puzzles, and even singing. They like to be read to, and their vocabulary is pretty good.

Francis couldn't read, and we were not sure exactly what he could hear. We could play patty cake with Francis, but not much of anything else."

"My favorite behavior was to twirl rapidly like a whirling dervish," said Francis. "I would stand in the middle of a room and begin spinning my whole body on tiptoe like a human top at a rapid speed until dizziness overcame me. I really enjoyed seeing the room spin around me in a blur, and I relished the dizziness that resulted. Even after I stopped spinning, the room would still seem to be spinning around me. I was so dizzy. I would perform other repetitive motions and play with my toys in odd ways. I was also unable to relate to other people or to express any emotions, give affection, or make friends. For a while after I came to the family, Mom and Dad were totally unable to figure out what was going on with me. My bizarre behaviors—whirling, spinning objects, making noises, staring into space, and my self-isolation—totally perplexed my family.

"My biggest most-puzzling problem was my lonely, self-absorbed behavior," relates Francis. "My inability to hear properly and communicate with the world led to my isolation and resulted in my displaying autistic tendencies. I withdrew into my own little world. My most visible tendencies were to make odd repetitive noises and gyrations."

Autistic? What on Earth is Autistic?

"My problems finally came to light when a friend of Mom was able to explain what was happening. At the Catholic church we attended, Mom had a friend who ran a special school for autistic children. Her name was Sarah Litch."

Recalled Sarah, "Francis was a new addition to Miss Kay's classroom in Martin Luther King Jr. Montessori Preschool in 1979. He was the center of attention, and Kay led the way in her positive, loving embrace of Francis as well as her open expectations for him. My son, Andy, was four years old and a classmate of Francis. Each day, Andy reported on not what he had done that morning but what Francis had accomplished.

"Across the street from Montessori preschool was the Catholic church where his parents were members as was my family. It was there that I learned of Betty and Bob Smith who had adopted ten children with difficulties. They were fierce advocates for each of them and loving parents to them all. Occasionally, I would get glimpses of Francis's growth and progress both at church and at the Montessori school. He, of course, was doing many things that he was never supposed to accomplish."

The family was at church one Sunday when Francis was acting out, staring, twirling, and using his fingers. Sarah Litch came over and said to Bob and Betty, "Are you aware that your son is autistic?"

"Autistic? What on earth is autistic?" Betty replied. "I'd never heard of it. No one else had either. All of our children had special needs, but none of them had what was called autistic." Before Francis was officially diagnosed, Betty was already one leap ahead in working with her son's newest battle.

"At this time, I was also the principal of a public school for exceptional children," Sarah reminisced. "We had a number of children with autism. I learned of the book *Son Rise* by Barry Neil Kaufman and Samahria Lyte Kaufman. I read the book in one weekend and immediately ordered fifteen copies for my staff and parents. I also gave a copy to the Smiths. Later, when I headed a private school where we had several children with autism, we sent staff to be trained by the Kaufmans. This book and the training at their home and center profoundly changed the way our staff worked successfully with autistic children. I am sure it had a profound effect on the way the Smith family viewed Francis and how they worked with him. Francis's parents had the wisdom and gift of understanding the techniques used."

Written in 1976, this is the story of a little boy named Raun, who from infancy lived in a peculiar world of his own due to autism. After he developed an ear infection as a baby, he developed bizarre autistic behaviors, rocking, spinning objects, zoning out, and rarely looked at or responded to people. He also did not talk. Raun's parents devised a one-on-one program to work with him and try to bring him out of himself. Their "classroom" was the bathroom because it had the least amount of distractions of any other place in the home. The whole family pitched in and worked with him in every activity he did and talked him through the entire day's activities. Little by little, he began to emerge from his solitary world with the help of his family's program.

Once Betty read *Son Rise*, her eyes were opened to Francis's struggles. Before knowing Sarah, she had never heard of autism. In *Son Rise*, she saw many of Raun's strange behaviors that were so similar to her son's. Like Raun, he had retreated into his own curious little world. He whirled like a dervish and spun plates and other round objects just as Raun did. For long lengths of time, he would tune out the world around him and just stare and stare, lost inside of his own world no one else could fathom. Inspired greatly by Raun's story, Betty began to painstakingly work with Francis, one on one.

"For example," said Francis, "Mom would talk me through the day's activities. As we went up or down stairs, Mom would say, 'Up, up, up' or 'Down, down, down,' to me. She would verbally describe to me everything we were doing together throughout the day. 'Up' became the first word I spoke. The goal was to immerse me in a world of human communication and eventually enable me to communicate on my own."

Another Daunting New Diagnosis

As a family, as they all did with one another, everyone pitched in to help Francis come out of his inner world. Slowly, his issues were addressed, one by one. Francis had to keep breathing through the tracheostomy until he was five years old. Aside from the immense full-time job of keeping his trach in top working order, it also kept him from entering society. Out in the brutal, hard, cold real world, he was kept out of preschool because teachers and children were afraid of his maladies and tubes. At last, after years of trying to convince his doctors it would be safe to do so, Dr. Singer—ear, nose, and throat doctor (ENT) at Riley Hospital—finally allowed the trach to be discontinued. Yet Francis's gavage feeding was not.

In an effort to wean Francis off the gavage feedings, Betty started to train him to take soft food and liquids by mouth with a baby spoon and sipper cup. The challenge was his severe large cleft palate and other deformities in his mouth. Betty never gave up. After a lengthy and determined effort, she was rewarded when her son was finally safely able to take food and liquid by mouth.

***

Francis's multiple maladies aside, what concerned Bob and Betty the most was his hearing. Since their child still could not speak, it was assumed he was deaf.

Bob and Betty vowed to do anything and everything in order to help their newest child move forward in life, just as they had with all their children. An audiologist was consulted. It was determined that what Francis needed was some type of bone conduction hearing aid, a device that would pick up the sounds around Francis and send them to a vibrating earpiece strapped to his temple where the sound energy would vibrate through the bone and into his inner ear.

"I remember my first bone conduction hearing aid," said Francis. "My audiologist led Mom and Dad to a headband-mounted hearing aid with a body-worn battery pack. It had a chrome body battery pack that took one AAA battery. A long cord connected it to a vibrating earpiece mounted on a headband to hold it against my right temple. This device finally opened me up to a world of sound. The hearing aid, by allowing me to hear for the first time ever, paved the way for my eventually learning to speak and communicate effectively during my early childhood. The hearing aid helped me get out of my autistic world that stemmed partially from my inability to hear. As I became able to hear with the aid, I began to emerge from my silent inner world and participate in the real world of sound and communication."

Francis Smith, youngster.

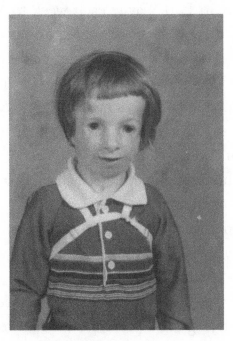

Francis at age six.

Teaching a Telephone Pole to Talk

After Francis's cleft palate was mostly closed, it was discovered that he had been able to somewhat hear all along through the opening. More surgery in the future would eventually be required to complete the closure, but for now, he was nearly completely deaf without his hearing aid.

The next goal the Smiths tackled was to teach Francis how to speak from scratch. Two years after the Smiths moved from New Haven to Garrett, Bob and Betty found out about a renowned speech therapist in Fort Wayne, Myra Conley. Myra enjoyed the distinct reputation of "teaching a telephone pole to talk." Betty wasted no time at all in taking Francis to Fort Wayne each week to Myra's home. Each speech therapy session lasted an hour or more, and most of that time was spent trying to get him to establish eye contact with Myra. Francis would just sit at the front of her desk kicking at her knees that was his way of communicating his impatience and frustration. The ever-patient Myra was not about to let him get the best of her, no matter what or how long it took, which only frustrated him even more.

Myra had turned her garage into a partial sitting room with a two-way mirror so parents could watch how she handled their children.

"Francis was not eating properly because of his cleft palate. I was trying to help them wean him from his feeding tube. He didn't like it, and he started kicking my knees, and boy, was he strong! I moved back and spread my knees apart so he couldn't kick my knees. He got so frustrated he bit the desk. I told him it wouldn't do him any good." For many years, Myra kept that desk with Francis's teeth marks permanently etched into it.

"After two years of not giving up on Francis, I had a huge breakthrough with him when he was about five," continued Myra. "Betty was standing in the doorway jiggling her keys. This was a habit of hers. Francis whipped his head around and looked right at her. Up until that time, we were all very unsure what—or if—Francis could hear because of all of his deformities. At that moment, I said to myself, 'Aha! You're mine now!'"

Myra, determined as she was, began to win Francis over, one step at a time. Slowly but surely, she began the arduous task of teaching him from the beginning. First, Francis had to learn to make simple speech sounds. Eventually, he progressed to single letters, then the alphabet, then simple words, phrases, and sentences. Steadily, he was transformed from a nonverbal child to one who could speak somewhat normally so that people close to him could understand him. Eventually, the funding ran out for his speech therapy just before he started kindergarten. It was difficult to no longer be able to continue, for Myra and the Smiths had formed a solid relationship, and she was considered a member of their family.

"To this day, we still keep in contact with her as a dear friend," stated Francis. "I credit Myra with giving me the gift of speech. Determined to make eye contact, she stuck with me until I finally made eye contact with her beyond my autistic world. Once she got my attention, she was able to work with me to build a vocabulary of speech sounds, then letters, then words, and finally complete sentences."

Reality Bites

I would say to them, "You are you, and God made you special."
—Betty Smith

***

In the heartland of America, as in the south, the early sixties and onward were still fraught with racial tensions and attitudes toward the challenged and people of color, a disheartening reality for Bob and Betty. Much to their alarm, they soon learned that a high-ranking member of the Ku Klux Klan lived only blocks away. Although they were personally never bothered, it wasn't something they could completely put out of their minds either. What did bother them were the neighbors that refused to speak to them. One neighbor went so far as to call her children terrible names. Doors closed in their faces, schools turned their children away, and people unabashedly openly stared and glared, causing her and the children great distress. Even some members of their local church they still attended shunned them as several of the children could not sit still in their pew for the sermons.

Betty sadly stated, "While some of the congregation lovingly reached out, the reality was the children weren't accepted very well. They couldn't deal with them, especially James and his terrible behavior." They decided to leave their church.

"My husband was raised and baptized in the Catholic church, and it was ingrained in him, so it was difficult for him to let go of that," remembered Betty. At the time of their decision, they had not chosen another church to attend. Once again, the Good LORD intervened, ironically through their son James.

James was their first biracial son who was born to an alcoholic, crack cocaine-addicted birth mother, and he would suffer the consequences of her terrible choices for the rest of his life. Betty found that her struggles with him were far different than those of her other children's. For one, he could only eat organic foods that were not readily accessible in those days, and she constantly had to be on guard to make sure he never ingested any food that contained food dye that was an ongoing recipe for disaster. He couldn't handle the chemicals because they set him off.

"What happened to James wasn't his fault," said Betty. "He had very little control over his own behavior that kept him out of schools."

James was constantly being sent home from school for his outbursts and disruptive behaviors. Finally, they were left with no other choice than to find him his own teacher for home schooling. Jenny was a gracious, patient young woman who immediately fell in love with James, as he did with her, which allowed their relationship to be a productive one.

***

One day, Jenny took James to the local fair. Bible Baptist Church (now Lakewood Park Baptist Church) had a booth there. A very lovely lady with a gracious demeanor leaned out and said to James, "Why are you playing hooky? Shouldn't you be in school?"

James replied, "Talk to my teacher. She's behind me."

Jenny was very excited by what she heard. Bible Baptist Church had a school, and from what she was hearing, James would be welcome. But the caveat was the school cost money. Jenny told Betty all about it when she brought James home, but Betty was disheartened because she knew they didn't have the money for the tuition. She silently prayed about the situation for the rest of the day before Bob got home. She didn't want to put any more stress on her husband who took on weekend work preparing taxes during tax season to make ends meet.

Betty's heartfelt prayer was answered even before Bob walked through the door.

"Guess what, Honey. I got a raise today," Bob happily announced. Betty was speechless.

When she recovered, she excitedly told Bob about the church school. Her husband's raise was just enough to cover not only the tuition for James but for the rest of their younger children as well.

"God is so good. Always," marveled Betty. "I've never seen the LORD not take a bad situation and turn it around for good. We relied heavily on Romans 8:28: 'And we know that all things work together for good to them that love God, to them who are called according to His purpose.'"

Immediately, the Smith family began attending Bible Baptist Church where they were met with open arms. Soon, church members dropped by to chip in. Betty found herself surrounded by loving people who offered their support. Their pastor's wife became a good friend, and in short order, their home held weekly Bible studies.

Still, racial tensions were reported practically daily on the news, so the television remained mostly off, which was fine with Betty. The children quickly found other ways to entertain themselves by playing games with one another or engaging in their latest musical instrument.

Hearts Full of Hate

Outside of her tightly knit circle, Betty found herself succumbing to the attitudes stares, finger pointing, and rude comments from their neighbors. For the most part, Bob ignored their rudeness, but still, it was the children they needed to protect. What Bob could not ignore was the toll the ongoing terrible rejection was taking on his wife. Betty was sinking into depression.

"We raised our children to be independent. We raised them to not acknowledge the color of their skin or their disabilities. I would say to them, 'You are you, and God made you special,'" recalled Betty, "and here we were faced with this." Society was saying something else entirely, and it was cruel. All she wanted to do was pack up her family and leave Garrett.

Bob's constant traveling did not help. Before the situation turned into a crisis, their faithful LORD intervened—again.

The Desire to Run

As winter slowly transitioned into spring, Bob and Betty thought how enjoyable it would be to build a large deck in the front of the house so the family could enjoy their meals outside when the weather was nice. Jimmy, their contractor, also had a landscaping business and was mildly learning disabled. He became quite a curiosity to the children who always surrounded him, asking questions while he worked. So he included them in any work they were able to do. It became a game as to who could pound the most nails in the fastest. The deck was built in no time.

Yet the turning point came later when Betty wanted a nice oak cabinet to be built in the downstairs bathroom. This time, Bob hired an African American man to do the honors. He and his wife were the only two African Americans for miles around in Garrett. By now, Betty was at the end of her rope with the attitude and meanness toward her family.

The gentleman, whose name Betty cannot remember, immediately captivated her with his kind and unassuming manner. The children all lit up and ran over to greet him as soon as he entered into their home. While he was building the cabinet, Betty changed her mind and told him the cabinet should be moved elsewhere. She said to him, "We won't be staying here much longer."

The gentleman stopped what he was doing, turned, and looked Betty straight in the eye. "Mrs. Smith," he said, "you're running. You best stay put. We wanted to run too, but we decided to stay, and now we are a very respected family here. You have your children to think about. They have enough challenges, and they need to learn to take a stand and get busy doing what God intended for them to do. Running won't do them any good. Only you can teach them that."

As stunned as Betty was, she said, "I told my husband, and he said, 'Honey, I kind of have to agree with that fellow.' We stayed for over thirty years."

Start children off on the way they should go,
and even when they are old they will not turn from it.
—Proverbs 22:6

Chapter 3

A Christmas Story
1980

For unto you is born
This day in the city of David,
A Savior,
Which is Christ the Lord.

—Luke 2:11

A Most Memorable Christmas—Part 1

Now that Francis was able to eat on his own and was able to hear and somewhat talk, Bob and Betty decided it was time to go visit Bob's uncle, Gene, and his wife Irma and his sister, Stewie, for Christmas so they could finally meet Francis.

Gene was a self-made, very wealthy dentist millionaire who lived in a beautiful mansion in Joliet, Illinois, which the Smiths had not yet seen. Irma, like Betty, had given birth to three stillborn children. Because of their uncertainty over adoption, they chose to remain childless. While Gene had his growing dental practice to occupy his time, his wife was a beautiful and popular top socialite and well-known artist. She also ran the gift store of Joliet's local hospital. They were known for giving substantial donations to the local junior college and hospital. They had invited the Smiths to stop and have Christmas lunch with them along the way to visit Bob's sister, Aunt Stewie, in Galesburg, Illinois, where they planned to spend the night.

The closer they got to Christmas, the more Betty was uncertain over their plans. The children were all challenged, which was difficult in a home that was not geared for difficulties, especially with Susie who battled cerebral palsy. Rob and Rebecca were both eating well after their own cleft palate surgeries, but they were still very shy and wary. Christopher's overall distrust made it difficult for him to reach out to others and spent his time as close to James as possible, who had his own behavior issues. Angel could be extremely outspoken at times, and Francis, of course, still had his tracheostomy. Plus, Betty had no idea how Gene and Irma celebrated Jesus's birth. The Smiths had deliberately kept their children away from the secular Christmas, meaning that Santa Claus, the elves, and the lively secular songs that ensued were never allowed in their home. The younger children were not even aware of them. Christmas in their home was the time the family celebrated the birth of Jesus, their LORD and Savior, and nothing else. Living on a tight budget did not leave room for Christmas shopping. Instead, each child pulled a name from a hat, then made a handmade gift for that person to express their love for them. It was a lovely time for all of them, so Betty had no idea what they were in for.

Immediately, the children went to work on handmade presents for Uncle Gene and Aunt Irma and for Aunt Stewie. They chose to build birdhouses for each of them, and for days, they excitedly drew the plans and started to build them using felt, glue, and popsicle sticks. As Betty lovingly watched, the children all contributed to the two works of art for three people they barely knew. Even Francis contributed, slapping on a popsicle stick or a piece of felt here and there. Bob and Betty were so proud of their children's original creations! All they could see was their beauty.

Who the Heck Is Santa Claus and Where Is Jesus?

It was so early Christmas Eve morning that dawn hadn't quite broken when the Smiths packed their brood into their station wagon for their trek from Indiana to Illinois. The only person missing was Edwin who had decided to spend Christmas with a friend of his from college. Peter was with them, and he was especially pleased that he was able to join the family. He recently began working at White's Institute and had fallen in love. His lovely girlfriend was also at White's Institute, and he was planning to propose marriage. Knowing he was going to ask her to marry him, he wanted to spend his last Christmas as a single man with his family. He was twenty years old.

"Peter was so well loved and accepted, and he worked so hard," recalls Betty. She and Bob could not have been prouder over how their beautiful boy had turned out.

Dawn didn't break until they were on the road from Indiana to Illinois. None of the younger children could sleep because they were so excited, so Bob turned on the radio to a Christian radio station where they heard the Word and sang Christmas carols. The children all knew "Away in the Manger," "Joy to the World," "Hark the Herald Angels Sing," and several others by heart. It was a delight when they all sang along. Caught in the joy of it all, even Francis joined in with his very cute utterings. The hours flew by, and everyone was filled with joy.

Almost from the first day that Francis joined the family, Angel, especially, had befriended him as her very own little brother, and their bonding was tight and fast. Nothing pleased her more than to be his big sister, but even she could not coax him away from the scenery they passed by. With his nose pressed against the window, Francis was enthralled by the outdoor Christmas displays that whizzed by along certain parts of the highway.

Around eleven o'clock in the morning, Bob said it was time to start looking for the turnoff. The singing quieted when Bob turned off the freeway.

Driving slowly through the neighborhood, they began to look for Uncle Gene and Aunt Irma's mansion. The children were silent and completely mesmerized by the opulent displays of festively decorated homes and their yards. Brightly lit larger-than-life Santa Clauses, reindeers, sleds, and snowmen adorned nearly every single front lawn, and the houses were outlined with beautiful colored lights. Even the trees on the front lawns were decorated. It was truly an amazing sight. Not one home was spared, and one had the impression that everyone was trying to outdo the other. Even Bob and Betty were speechless! What was conspicuous by its absence was the nativity. There wasn't one anywhere.

Susie piped up, "Who is that old man with the white beard?"

"That's Santa Claus," mumbled Angel.

"Who is Santa Claus?" retorted Susie.

"It doesn't matter," Angel sighed. "He isn't real; he's just colorful."

"Where's Jesus?" said Susie.

"I guess they forgot about Him," Angel sadly replied.

Let the Show Begin!

Bob turned onto a street that was even more opulent than the others. "We're here, kids. This is the street." Bob pulled in to a brightly lit driveway.

The children were silent, their eyes as big as saucers. Uncle Gene's mansion was the most abundantly decorated of all. It even had copper gutters! A brightly lit, quite larger-than-life Santa sat in his oversized sleigh filled with artfully wrapped presents, all pulled by giant reindeer. The entire front of the house, even the windows and doors, were out-lined by dangling white icicle lights, and the outdoor trees bore blinking colored lights! Bob and Betty exchanged "uh-oh" glances. The children couldn't take their eyes off the enormous festive display.

No sooner did Bob and Betty open the car doors than the front door opened, and out came Uncle Gene and Aunt Irma, dressed as Santa and Mrs. Santa.

"Ho! Ho! Ho! Merry Christmas!" bellowed Uncle Gene. Aunt Irma looked rather pert herself as Mrs. Santa.

"Merry Christmas to you, Gene and Irma," Bob said. "Come on, kids, let's go inside and get warm. Peter, do you have Uncle Gene and Aunt Irma's gift?"

"Yes, Dad," Peter replied. He held the wrapped home-made birdhouse in his arms.

Quietly, the children gathered themselves together, none of them saying a word. Susie struggled as best she could, walking the distance in the cold, her braces freezing and her crutches sliding. She didn't dare try to walk without her aids. Angel held Francis's hands. James held his lunch pail in one hand and Christopher's hand in the other. The entry hallway of the mansion was decorated in such a way that the outdoors appeared to continue on inside the house. Christmas lights were wrapped around the bannister, and to the left was the large nine-foot beautifully decorated, brightly lit Christmas tree that stood in front of the massive picture window. Under the tree were dozens of beautiful ornately wrapped Christmas presents. Across the room, more colored lights were strewn across a massive brick fireplace that glowed and crackled with a log fire, spewing its warmth to every corner of the room. Irma took their coats and James's lunch pail and handed them to their African American house couple that stood at attention behind her. Betty winced. Irma ushered them into the living room where two couches and easy chairs were gathered near the fireplace. Irma quickly situated herself at the upright organ that was next to the fireplace. The children were speechless, having no idea what was going on. Bob and Betty were both skeptical of what was to happen next.

"Let's all get in the spirit. Let's sing Christmas songs!" He turned to Aunt Irma. "Hit it, Mrs. Claus!"

Irma expertly glided over the organ keys. Out came "Jingle Bells." Since none of the children knew the words to the song, they sat politely on the couches, each of them looking around with confused wonder at the rather outrageous display around them. Bob and Betty sat motionless in the chairs, joining in the best they could. A couple of the older children tried to follow their lead. At least, their lips moved.

"Let's sing 'Santa Baby'!" You all know that one, don't you?"

Nope.

After a rousing rendition of "Santa Baby" that Gene and Irma sang only to each other, the singing stopped.

"Well," Gene said, "so much for Christmas songs."

Bob piped in, "I'm afraid they don't know these songs, Gene. They only know Christmas carols. The children have never celebrated anything other than the birth of Jesus. They don't understand who Santa Claus is either."

"In that case, maybe Santa Claus should introduce himself." Betty shifted uncomfortably. "That will brighten them up." He left the room briefly then returned with a large burlap sack, brimming with presents, slung across his shoulder.

"Ho! Ho! Ho! Merry Christmas!" Uncle Gene bellowed. "Now you'll all know who Santa Claus is!" Uncle Gene took two beautifully wrapped packages out and looked at the tags. "Well, well, well," he said. He leaned over toward Angel with her gift in his hand. "Tell me, young lady, have you been naughty or nice?"

Angel, flustered, looked to both her parents.

Bob spoke up, "All of our children are very nice, Uncle Gene."

"Isn't that great to know, Mrs. Claus? Here you are, young lady." He handed Angel her present. "Well, let's pass out the rest of the presents, shall we, Mrs. Claus?" Aunt Irma was delighted. Together, they passed each present out to the proper name bearer. Once everyone had their presents, Uncle Gene told them to open them. All the children received Uncle Gene and Aunt Irma's signature practical gifts. They each received a beautiful carved wood pencil box filled with wood pencils engraved with each of their names.

"Gene and Irma were very practical and frugal people," remembered Betty. "They always wanted the children to have what they needed for their education."

Francis was very happy and quite content with the colorful wrapping paper, and he hadn't even gotten to the pencil box. The rest of the children said, "Thank you," and were truly pleased with their gifts. Bob received a brand-new Dopp Kit complete with the finest razor, comb, and soaps; and Betty received a top-of-the-line new steam iron.

"I picked it myself. I thought you could use it." Irma winked.

"I've never seen a finer iron in my life," praised Betty. "We have a present for you."

"Let's go have lunch first," said Uncle Gene. "Then Irma and I will open our gift." Before Irma could respond, Uncle Gene was leading the way into the dining room where the table was beautifully set with sterling, china, and crystal, something the children rarely saw. Bob and Betty exchanged glances and got the children settled at the table. Boy, this was no time for a lesson in manners. Francis was deeply enchanted by the silverware, and no sooner had Betty gotten herself seated next to him when he dropped his soupspoon on the floor. In less than a second, Mr. Bailey picked up the soupspoon, placed it on a silver tray, turned, and headed toward the kitchen. Mrs. Bailey stood stone-faced, staring straight dead ahead. A moment later, Mr. Bailey returned with a clean soupspoon and placed in back on the table in its rightful place. Next, the fork was on the floor. Betty was mortified. Again, Mr. Bailey appeared with the silver tray. Bob stopped him in his tracks.

"Mr. Bailey, why don't you just put the fork back on the table please." Mr. Bailey did as he was asked. His jaw was clearly clenching.

Uncle Gene sat at one end of the large dining room table, and Aunt Irma sat the other end. Gene picked up a bell and rang it. Everyone stopped talking and gave Uncle Gene their rapt attention.

"Our couple, Mr. and Mrs. Bailey, spent all day yesterday and this morning cooking this glorious meal that Irma planned for this wonderful occasion," said Gene proudly. He turned toward his wife. "What's on the menu, Dear?"

"Crab bisque with a dollop of sherry, for starters." Betty turned white. Bob clenched his jaw. "Followed by stuffed game hens, croissants, peas in wine cream sauce, and wild rice soufflé," she announced proudly.

Betty kicked Bob under the table. He kicked her back. *Oh no.* Francis's silverware was spread across the carpet, and he was now enamored with the crystal salt and pepper shakers; and lunch hadn't even started. Mr. Bailey picked up the silverware and placed it back on the table. Mrs. Bailey stoically served the soup and crackers. Mr. Bailey followed with the sherry. James sat at his place staring at his china plates.

"Why don't you hold off on the sherry for the children, Mrs. Bailey, if you don't mind," Betty politely mentioned. Mr. Bailey bypassed the children then on to the adults with the sherry.

***

Betty continued, "Uh, Irma, James is on a very special diet. May he have his lunch pail please."

"Yes, of course. Mrs. Bailey, would you clear this young man's plate and bring his own lunch out for him please?"

Within moments, James had his sandwich and bowl of applesauce in front of him all served on china.

Gene raised his wine glass. "Merry Christmas, everyone! Let's dig in!"

Bob interrupted. "Let's say a Christmas blessing first, Gene. The children never eat without saying the blessing first."

Everyone took one another's hands. Bob began the family prayer. "LORD, thank you for this beautiful Christmas Eve Day where we celebrate the birth of your son Jesus, our wonderful Savior. LORD, please bless Gene and Irma who so graciously opened their home for us on this special day and Mr. and Mrs. Bailey who are so graciously serving us. We love you, LORD. Please bless this food to our bodies. Amen."

Betty mouthed a silent prayer. "Please, LORD, get us through this meal."

Plop! Francis dropped his soupspoon directly into the soup bowl that splashed all over the white silk tablecloth. Mrs. Bailey hurried over to remove the bowl. Mr. Bailey followed with a cloth. Betty leaned over. "Mrs. Bailey, why don't we just skip the soup for Francis. I'm afraid he's a bit young to eat soup properly." Mrs. Bailey did as she was asked with a serious look of disapproval on her face.

The children were even more challenged with the stuffed game hens that only managed to slide all over the plate, knocking the rest of the food all over the table and themselves. Susie, especially, had a very difficult time. Neither Betty nor Bob were sure if the children even ate the food. The situation was hopeless. Thankfully, Irma and Gene, who were always so gracious, pretended not to notice.

As the last of the dinner was cleared away and cleaned up as much as possible, Irma announced it was time for coffee, cocoa, and Christmas cookies. China dessert plates, coffee cups and cocoa mugs, and fresh silverware arrived. Mrs. Bailey came to the table with a tray of perfect, elegantly decorated Christmas cookies and festively decorated petite fours. Betty turned to her and said, "Mrs. Bailey, why don't you place the tray on the table. It is much easier if the children can help themselves."

Susie said out loud exactly what Betty was thinking. "Are we supposed to eat these?"

By now, Betty was beyond horrified; she just wanted it over. Mrs. Bailey was rather indignant at this point and did nothing but let the children make their messes. Mr. Bailey, expressionless, followed with coffee and cocoa for the children.

"Oh please, LORD, let this meal be over," prayed Betty silently. Bob, at least, was engaged in an animated conversation with his brother while Betty and Irma tried to chat while she attempted to keep one eye on the children. Finally, the last drops of coffee and cocoa were finished.

A Gift Straight from the Heart

Bob stood up from the table. "It looks like we'll have to push off pretty soon. As soon as we get cleaned up, we'd like to present our gift to you." The children rose and headed for the nearest bathrooms, followed by Betty. When they returned, Bob, Gene, and Irma were sitting around the kitchen table.

"Look how nice everyone cleaned up," Irma said when the children and Betty returned.

"Peter, why don't you get Uncle Gene and Aunt Irma's gift?" reminded Bob. "It's in the living room." A few moments later, Peter appeared with the rather original childlike wrapped present. He placed it on the kitchen table.

Gene looked at his wife. "Why don't you do the honors, Dear?" Excitedly, Irma opened the gift. The wrapping nearly fell away on its own, leaving the homemade birdhouse fully displayed. Betty beamed, and Bob and the children waited silently.

"Do you like it?" piped up Angel.

"Of course, I do," replied Irma happily. "I've always wanted one."

Gene leaned over and whispered into his wife's ear, "What is it?"

Irma whispered back, "I have no idea."

Betty could tell Irma had no idea what it was, and neither did Gene. "It took the children nearly a week to design and make this very special birdhouse from scratch, just for you," Betty remarked proudly.

"Oh, how lovely. It's a beautiful birdhouse, isn't it, Gene?" He nodded with the same happy but perplexed look as his wife. "We can hang it right outside our kitchen window so Uncle Gene can watch the birds in the morning."

"That's exactly where it will go. How did you know we liked birds so much?" Gene jovially inquired. "Bailey must have informed you. Right, Bailey?"

Mr. Bailey didn't say one word. The look on Mrs. Bailey's face was frozen.

Beautifully Wrapped Emptiness

As they gathered in the entryway to receive their belongings, Peter peeked into the living room at all the wrapped Christmas gifts under the tree. "You sure have a lot of Christmas gifts left, Uncle Gene. Are you having more visitors today?"

"Oh no," he replied. "Those boxes are empty. They're just for show." The children looked quizzical but didn't say a word.

The family said their goodbyes next to the car. "You drive safely; it's pretty icy out there," reminded Gene.

"Bob is an excellent driver. Thank you so much for such a lovely Christmas afternoon, Gene and Irma," said Betty. "We'll pray for special blessings for your New Year."

"Thank you," Gene and Irma replied in unison.

As soon as the family was settled in the car, Betty whispered under her breath, "Thank you, LORD, that Gene and Irma were so gracious and that they finally got to see the children again and meet Francis. Amen."

Getting settled inside the car, Bob leaned in toward Betty. "I think we're going to have a lot of explaining to do," he said.

Before they left the driveway, Bob led his family in prayer. "Dear LORD, please guide and protect us as we continue on our journey. We ask that you bless Gene and Irma, and please, LORD, our prayer is that in some way they were introduced to You and Your Son, Jesus. Amen."

"Amen," followed the others.

Gene and Irma waved as they pulled out of the driveway. Everyone waved back.

As soon as Bob started to drive down the street, one of the children burst forth in song. "Jingle Bells, fat man smells..."

Betty's neck snapped toward the back seat. "What?! Which one of you did that?"

The children all stared innocently at her, none of them giving her any clue as to who the guilty party was.

"Don't let me hear that again." She gave them a stern look, then turned her attention back to the front. The children stifled their giggles.

Back on the freeway, the children were quiet as they pondered their rather-different afternoon. All the children admired their personalized pencils and boxes. Francis was intrigued by his, but for his own reasons.

Christopher complained, "I'm hungry." Several of the other children joined in.

"Hang in there, kids. I'm sure Aunt Stewie has something wonderful for us to eat waiting for us at her house," reminded Betty.

After a short period of silence, Susie piped up, "Where was Jesus? Why wasn't he there?"

"I don't think He was invited," observed Peter.

"We'll have to pray for them about that," said Angel.

A Memorable Christmas—Part 2

During the shorter ride to Galesburg, the Smiths were subdued as each of them contemplated their visit with Uncle Gene and Aunt Irma. Betty and Bob were as worn-out as the children were. Even the radio was turned off, and it was so quiet you could hear a pin drop. Betty was thinking she knew Stewie was a devoted Catholic who loved the LORD Jesus with all her heart. There was no doubt in Betty's mind that Stewie would be celebrating the birth of Jesus.

Aunt Stewie was the secretary for the president at Knox College in Galesburg, Illinois. She was the same age as Betty and permanently single, which back then was a bit of an oddity. Asked once why she never married, she boldly replied that she was far too particular about the man she would marry, and he didn't exist.

"I'm not like you, Betty, who married the first guy who came along," joked Stewie.

"What?" Betty was shocked until Stewie started to laugh.

Betty's relationship with Stewie had not always been close. Many years before when they were first getting to know each other, Stewie wasn't quite enamored with Betty. During one of their earlier visits, Betty had been soaking in the bathtub when Stewie marched in the bathroom without knocking and threw a handful of detergent into the bathtub, announcing, "I don't want you to leave a ring in the tub," before she turned and marched right back out. Betty nearly flew out of the bathtub because the detergent began to sting. Over the years, their relationship gradually softened as they learned to respect each other's differences and life choices. Now their relationship was strong as the two women genuinely enjoyed each other's company.

Aunt Stewie was very well-known in her own right. Aside from her coveted secretarial position, model-esque figure and flawless face, she was a fashionista who had a wardrobe that was the envy of everyone around her. A fantastic musician, vocalist, and actress, she appeared regularly in local theatre, and she was the envy of everyone who knew her. Boy, oh, boy, did she love to throw parties. What Betty came to learn for certain was that Stewie was even more beautiful on the inside than she was on the outside.

The entire Smith family adored her. Every Christmas, Stewie made matching pajamas for the entire family along with a handmade Christmas ornament that she sent to them. Without fail, she called on Christmas morning where she made sure she spoke with all the children. The family rarely saw her in person, and this was the first time she would be meeting Francis.

Some of the younger children were fast asleep in the back of the station wagon. A few miles from Aunt Stewie's home, Betty turned around to announce they were almost there and for everyone to straighten up. The older ones helped the younger ones get ready.

The evening was black and clear, glimmering with brilliant stars that appeared to touch the earth. Finally, Bob found Stewie's private road and turned on to it. Both Bob and Betty were perplexed as to why the road was packed with cars.

"There must be a big party going on around here. I hope we can find a place to park nearby," sighed Betty.

"It's Christmas Eve, Dear," replied Bob.

Bob drove slowly, looking for a parking space. Oh my goodness! The party was at Stewie's house! Through the large picture windows, they could see women in dresses and men in suits enjoying themselves with the wonderful and tasteful Christmas decorations in the background. They were stunned. Just then, Stewie rushed outside to greet them.

"Over here! I saved the best parking spot just for you. Hi, kids!" Stewie waved to the kids. Some of them waved back. "I hope you don't mind, but I've invited a few friends over to meet you and the kids. Don't worry about bringing your stuff in. I'll get someone to help you."

A couple of elegantly dressed women joined Stewie beside the car. One of them peeked through Bob's open window. "Oh, look at them! They're all so cute!"

Bob and Betty were speechless. The children had never been shown off before, and she had no way of knowing how these strangers, let alone the children, would react. For a moment, she was terrified until Bob nudged her. He gave her a look of assurance that everything would be all right.

Slowly, all the kids got out of the car where Aunt Stewie greeted them with great big hugs. Stewie nudged her friends. "Go on up and tell them they're here." The women went ahead.

"Stewie," said Bob, "we certainly didn't expect this. We thought—"

Betty continued, "Our children have never experienced a room full of strangers—"

"You have nothing to worry about. These are wonderful people, and they can't wait to meet you," replied Stewie. "I've told them all about you. Come on everyone, let's go inside."

"Let everyone put on their best smiles and best manners," Bob said. The children did as they were told. Betty felt as though they were all lambs going to the slaughter. Christopher practically crawled into James's arms.

Behold, I stand at the door, and knock: If any man
hear my voice, and open the door, I will come in to
him, and will sup with him, and he with me.

—Revelation 3:20

Inviting Jesus In

The front door opened. Immediately in their line of sight was a simple but gorgeously decorated Christmas tree with a large beautiful nativity scene displayed in front of it in all its glory. It took their breath away. Now *this* was Christmas!

In moments, the smiling guests surrounded the Smiths. Finally, it was Francis who broke the ice. One of the ladies wore a rhinestone charm bracelet that caught his attention, and right away, he reached out and grabbed her wrist so he could fixate on it more closely. The woman did not attempt to pull her arm away. In fact, she appeared amused by his action. Betty explained to her that he was autistic, and he liked her bracelet.

"Autistic? I never heard of it. How unusual." She took Betty by the elbow and steered them aside while Francis was pulled along, clinging tightly to her wrist. "Oh, please tell me all about it. He is sooooo cute!" she gushed. Betty, in her travel clothes and with a glass of champagne in hand, engaged in the subject, going into great depth.

Right away, each of the children had a new adult friend. Actually, most enjoyed the attention. Peter was talking to someone about White's Institute and his future plans. James spoke to another couple while Susie managed to stand upright on her crutches beside him. Rob and Rebecca allowed everyone to notice their strong resemblance with smiles on their faces. Christopher, for some baffling reason and much to the shock of his parents, managed to open up enough to enjoy the couple that was talking to him. They had all dropped their guard and were enjoying this unexpected good time.

Stewie whispered into Betty's ear, "You all must be hungry. I fixed a light buffet for everyone, so let's step into the dining room so everyone can have something to eat. You and the children go first." Stewie got everyone's attention, and the party gravitated to the dining room where the most scrumptious, elegant food spread awaited them. There was roast beef, Yorkshire pudding, baked salmon, mashed potatoes, a huge salad, butter rolls, green beans, and much more. So much for a "light" buffet!

Soon, everyone was gathered around the grand piano singing Christmas carols that the children loved and didn't hesitate to join in. It was a joyous evening for them all. But it was late, and the younger children were fading. The party broke up as Bob and Betty excused themselves to get their children off to bed. This was a Christmas no one in the family was ever going to forget.

A Very Special Christmas Blessing

Bob and Betty woke up to the sounds of Christmas morning and the delightful aroma of coffee and Stewie's gourmet cooking. Hurriedly, they put on their bathrobes and rushed downstairs.

As soon as Bob and Betty appeared, the children all rushed into the living room where their presents miraculously appeared overnight by the tree.

"Oh, thank goodness, you're finally up." Stewie laughed. She was wearing a pair of bright red-and-green flannel pajamas with a fluffy white bathrobe. "I couldn't contain them for another minute!"

While the adults stood with steaming cups of fresh coffee in their hands, they all delighted in the children who were excitedly unwrapping their new sets of hand-sewn jammies and white bathrobes. Of course, they wanted to put theirs on. Bob and Betty unwrapped their presents next. Their pajamas and robes matched their children's and Stewie's. They all went upstairs to change.

As soon as everyone came back down, all dressed in their matching pajamas, the children rushed straight to the table where Stewie had laid out a glorious Christmas breakfast in the formal dining room with its incredible spread of gourmet delights: bacon, ham, sausage, toast, eggs, coffee cake, cinnamon rolls, juice, and milk. There was plenty of "safe" food for James.

"Whoa! Hold your horses! Haven't we forgotten something?" Bob laughed.

The children stopped, grabbed hands, and stood with their heads bowed.

"That's better." Bob bowed his head. "Dear God, please bless this day as we celebrate the birth of your son, Jesus. Please bless Aunt Stewie and her wonderful home that is always filled with her love for you. We thank you, LORD, for the safe journey you have given us. In your name, we pray. Amen." The kids were twitching with excitement. "Okay, *now* you can eat!" Stewie started to laugh.

Sitting around the kitchen table, everyone was in a delightful mood. The children all felt very much at home, and they were behaving like it. They laughed and chattered away—all of them joined in!

"I hope you didn't mind the party I had for you last night. I've told so many of my friends about your amazing family, and when I told them you were coming for

Christmas, they nearly ganged up on me, asking to meet you! I couldn't possibly not invite them," she said.

Bob chuckled. "I have to tell you, Stewie, we just about had a heart attack when we saw so many people through the windows."

Betty laughed. "It was quite a shock. I was ready to turn around and go home. We had no idea. But I have to admit, we all had a wonderful time. Your friends were so taken with the children."

Angel piped up, "Look." She pointed to the handmade birdhouse they had made beautifully displayed, hanging from a tree in front of the kitchen window.

"It's so beautiful!" exclaimed Stewie. "I can't wait to show it off. I know the birds will love it when they come back this spring. Did all of you make it together?"

The children nodded.

"Marvelous! I will treasure this wonderful gift forever. I feel so special." The children beamed.

After breakfast, the table was cleared with help from the children. What amused them most was Aunt Stewie threw away the pan!

"It's old. I don't need it anymore," Aunt Stewie explained.

"Don't get any ideas, children." Betty laughed. "I'll have to keep an eye on our pots and pans for a while now."

The rest of the visit went so well. After changing clothes, several of the children went outside to throw snowballs. It was a wonderland outside! The others stayed in and quietly played with one of the games Stewie gave to them. The day passed by quickly, and after a simple meal, the family gathered around the tree and nativity for prayer time and to give thanks. Stewie played Christmas carols on the piano, and they all joined in. The day was all about Jesus. Finally, it was time for bed. The children loved Aunt Stewie, and none of them wanted to leave in the morning. Stewie extended the invitation to stay for another day or two, but Bob had to return home for some projects that were waiting for him at the house before he went back to his heavy travel schedule.

The next morning started very early. After a quick breakfast, it was time to leave. Stewie stood in the driveway wrapped in a heavy coat, waving goodbye with tears in her eyes.

Around the corner, Bob asked everyone if they had had a good time.

"The best!" said Angel.

"Now that was Christmas," said Betty softly.

Betty glanced in the rearview mirror. Christopher, their quiet son, had his nose pressed against the window. He was staring at Aunt Stewie's house as it disappeared around the corner. He was smiling!

The Word became flesh and made His dwelling among us. We have seen His glory, the glory of the one and only Son, who came from the Father, full of grace and truth.
—John 1:14

Chapter 4

A Test of Faith
1981–1982

*The dark moments of our life will last only as long as is
necessary for God to accomplish his purpose in us.*
—Charles Stanley

The Ever-faithful LORD

By now, the Smith household had dwindled down
to six children, but that had little impact on the constant
whirlwind of activity.

Francis had completed preschool at the Montessori
school in Fort Wayne. Now, with great excitement, he was
getting ready to attend kindergarten in Garrett, at J. E.
Ober Elementary School for the 1981–1982 school year.
Francis would be participating in Mrs. Hampshire's reading readiness class for part of each day. Bob and Betty had
heard many wonderful things about Mrs. Hampshire and
her reading readiness class that was specifically for children

who were in kindergarten and first grade who needed a little extra push like he did.

Just as had been expected, Francis and Mrs. Hampshire formed an instant friendship. She doted on him, and he adored her. For the first part of the morning, they worked together in the privacy of the hallway where his desk had been moved. For the rest of the day, Francis was in the regular kindergarten class. He loved being in class, and this was where he finally began to blossom.

Now that Francis was seven years old and out of kindergarten, he was facing two surgeries back to back in the summer of 1982. The first was to complete the repair of his fistula (hole in his cleft palate). The surgeon would close his cleft palate by temporarily sewing his tongue flap to the roof of his mouth for two weeks. The second stage required that his jaw be surgically split in two, realigned, then wired shut for two months. This procedure would take place at St. Louis Children's Hospital at the Washington University Medical Center, nearly four hundred miles away. His physician, Dr. Jeffrey Marsh, was the founder and medical director of the Craniofacial Deformities Institute. Since Riley Hospital for Children in Indianapolis did not have a craniofacial team, the doctors there had recommended the Smiths transfer to Dr. Marsh in St. Louis for Francis's complex craniofacial care from then on.

While Betty and Angel prepared Francis for the long trip to St. Louis and the even longer hospital stays, Bob made the preparations for the insurance for the hospitalization and medical needs. Out of their own pockets, he needed to make the arrangements for the back-and-forth travel, food, gas, and lodging. Since Angel intended to stay in St. Louis with Francis for the entire time, plans also had to be made for her accommodations. Betty's purpose was to be at home when Bob was traveling, then to go back to St. Louis as soon as Bob returned. Bob proposed to somewhat curtail as much of his own heavy travel schedule as he could in order to be home with the family as much as possible while Betty was away. Peter and Edwin, the two oldest children who no longer lived at home, made arrangements to help care for the household. Everything had to be executed down to the minutest detail.

In the midst of this came an unexpected surprise. Peter announced his engagement! Both he and his bride-to-be, who was also a graduate of White's Institute and now worked there, were so well thought of they were asked to become house parents after they married. The Smiths were beside themselves with excitement, and they couldn't wait to meet their future daughter-in-law. Betty was already mentally planning the wedding and for her future role as a mother-in-law even though the wedding was at least a year away. The Smiths were in a whirl just thinking about getting through this year!

On the morning of the surgery, Francis was as excited as he was nervous. Betty and Angel bid their tearful farewells as he was wheeled away from them on his gurney. Deeply medicated, he was lost in the world of gleaming stainless-steel cabinets, shiny surgical instruments, and strong overhead lights that faded in and out with the strength of his medication. The medical team was all dressed from head to toe in blue gowns, masks, and caps. The room was freezing! Francis was captivated by his surroundings, all the while feeling unsettled by pangs of nerves. The last thing he remembered was choosing strawberry as the flavor for his anesthesia mask that quickly engulfed him.

There are neither dreams nor any sense of time while under anesthesia. The next thing Francis hazily remembered were his mother and sister peering closely into his face. Much to his horror—and immediately noticeable—his tongue was sewn to the roof of his mouth! Thankfully, the nurse was expecting such a reaction, and she was there to administer something to calm his nerves. Not long afterward, he was wheeled into the intensive care unit where he was aware of other children who were all hooked up to oxygen and IV tubes. For the next two days, he was under constant observation.

A few days later, Francis was allowed to take liquid, fed to him by a syringe. It certainly was tricky learning to swallow with his tongue sewn to the roof of his mouth! Knowing that Francis was past the worst and was doing well, Betty left to make the hours-long trek back to Indiana.

Shortly after Betty left, Francis derailed the calm. While he was sleeping, he somehow managed to pry his tongue loose with his fingers. Thank the LORD, he was still under close observation because blood spewed everywhere! By the time he was wheeled back into surgery, he had lost over a pint of blood. Along with having his tongue reattached to the roof of his mouth, he was given a blood transfusion.

This time when he awoke, his hands were tied to the rails of his hospital bed. For Francis, that was the most unnerving aspect of his recovery.

Thankfully, the two weeks between surgeries sped by quickly. For the second phase of the surgery, Francis's jaw was to be split in two; then bone grafts, screws, and plates would be used to realign his jaw in a forward direction that would enable a more normal eating and speaking motion. Another positive outcome of having his jaw realigned was that he would now have a chin. This second phase of the surgery was expected to be far more daunting than the first part had been, but in typical Francis fashion, he simply rolled with the punches. Besides, he reveled in the non-stop attention. For the next two months, he would have to endure blenderized liquid food fed to him through a syringe, all the while with his tracheostomy tube in place. The first night of the second surgery was spent back in the intensive care unit (ICU). The next morning, he was released to spend the upcoming week in the ward. During that time, Francis progressed so well Dr. Marsh made the decision to allow him to return home to his family for the next two months of his recovery.

Coming Home to the Unexpected

To celebrate Francis's early homecoming, several members of the family—Bob, Betty, Angel, and James—arrived in St. Louis for the monumental event. Not everyone could fit into the station wagon, so Peter, Becky, Rob,

Edwin, and Christopher remained at home. The station wagon was jam-packed with Francis's medical supplies, but somehow, Bob, Betty, Angel, James, and Francis all managed to fit inside. While some of them managed to doze on and off during the all-night drive, Francis was able to sleep for nearly the entire time.

Dawn was perhaps a half hour away from breaking when the station wagon pulled into the garage in the back alley. Immediately noticeable and much to Bob and Betty's chagrin, the entire house was lit up, each and every room in the house! Bob mentioned something about the electric bill as Betty focused on getting the kids awake. Angel was the next to notice as she struggled to get Francis to sit up.

"What are all the lights doing on?" Angel complained. Bob stood in the driveway and frowned.

Edwin was the first to come outside, followed by Rob and Becky, then Christopher. Betty took one look at them and froze. Instead of pajamas, they were all fully clothed, and all of them were crying! Protectively, Angel let Francis stay in the car for a moment.

Bob spoke first, "What's wrong?"

Panicked, Betty blurted out, "Where's Peter?" Angel grabbed her hand.

Edwin spoke through sobs, "The police have been trying to find you. Peter was in an accident."

Angel let out a sob. Betty flew into Bob's arms, screaming. "No! No!"

Lights popped on in other houses as the neighbors peeked through curtains.

Bob hugged his wife tightly as he spoke calmly, "Edwin, is Peter alive?" Edwin barely nodded.

Bob continued, "Is he in the hospital?"

Edwin sobbed, "He's in Lutheran Hospital." Edwin paused before he went on, "A car hit him head-on."

Betty let out a hysterical shriek. Bob tried to gather her into his arms, but in her despair, she fought him. He grasped her into a bear hug and held her tightly, trying to calm her. Finally, she was quieted but still sobbing.

Bob gathered all the family together in the driveway, leading them in prayer for Peter, asking that the LORD's will be done in this tragic situation.

Every Parent's Nightmare

Nothing could prepare Bob and Betty for the excruciating, agonizing scene that awaited them. Inside the ICU, Peter lay unresponsive, in a coma on the hospital bed, swathed from head to toe in bandages. Eerily, the only sounds they could hear were the beeping and hissing of the life support machines that reminded them that they were what was keeping their son alive. Before they could even make it to the side of Peter's bed, they fell into each other's arms, each holding the other up, as they sobbed and sobbed.

The doctor in charge joined them inside the small cubicle, but it was several moments before Bob and Betty even noticed him. In his hands was Peter's chart. As gently as he could, the doctor explained that Peter had suffered a massive head trauma. "Peter is brain-dead, and there is no hope for recovery. Even if he does regain consciousness, he will be a vegetable for the rest of his life. The most difficult decision you will have to make is when you decide to take Peter off the respirator."

Neither Bob nor Betty was able to respond to the doctor. Grief-stricken, all they could do was stare blankly. Words just wouldn't come out. There were so many bandages and tubes coming out of him they couldn't even find his hand so they could hold on to him.

"Why?" Betty wailed. "Why?" Peter's future had looked so bright! He had overcome so much in his young life, and he had even found the young girl he planned to marry. No. No! This couldn't be happening!

Slowly, Bob and Betty regained their composure. Bob, especially, never questioned the LORD, not even now. Through his own heartbreak that even he couldn't understand in this moment, he trusted in the LORD completely, and he had to lead the family to move forward in faith. The tragic day ahead of them was going to be excruciating. They held hands as they prayed by Peter's bedside, talking to him and sobbing while asking the LORD for wisdom as to when to set Peter free. They both agreed they didn't want the other children there for his passing, but they did want them to come say goodbye to their beloved brother. Bob phoned Edwin and told him the tragic news. Edwin promised to bring the children to Peter's bedside as quickly as he could.

Francis remembers Peter lying perfectly still, wrapped from head to toe in bandages, with tubes and wires that were connected to noisy, beeping, hissing machines sticking out of him. *How could Peter sleep through all that noise?* he thought to himself. Mercifully for Francis, his youth and autism did not allow him to fully compute the gravity of the situation. Peter was special to him, as he was the one who chipped in the most to help with the very complex gavage feedings when Francis first arrived at the Smiths'. Their bond remained especially strong even after Peter no longer lived at the house. The family gathered in grief around Peter's bed. Each of the children professed their love for him, shared their fondest memory, and kissed him goodbye. Angel stayed steadfastly by Francis's side.

After Edwin left to go back home with the children, Bob and Betty stayed by Peter's side until they felt ready to ask the doctor to take him off the respirator. They grasped Peter's bandaged hands while they prayed, sang, and waited for the LORD to take their son home. Mercifully, they knew for certain that Peter had asked Jesus to be his personal LORD and Savior, so they had no doubts that he was going to go straight into the arms of Jesus. After all, they had God's promise, 2 Corinthians 5:8: "We are confident, I say, and willing rather to be absent from the body and, to be present with the Lord." In His graciousness, the LORD did not tarry. Peter peacefully passed into eternity.

Days later, the funeral home was packed. Bob and Betty held up the best they could while some of their children held up better than others. Peter's devastated, heartbroken fiancée arrived and introduced herself to Bob and Betty before falling into Betty's arms. Clinging to each other, the two women sobbed. Peter's loss hit everyone who knew him very, very hard.

Francis stood by Peter's casket, fixated on his beloved brother who was dressed in his favorite suit and his wide shirt collar open, reposed in a beautiful metallic box with a fluffy interior. Already, he named the casket the "dying trunk" because it resembled the trunk in which Susie carried her belongings off to college. The room was filled with flowers and cards.

Uncannily, Angel always knew what Francis was trying to process. She saw the questions in his eyes as he touched the casket. She leaned down and gently explained, "This isn't really Peter. This is just his earthly body that is going to be buried." What she said seemed to raise even more questions. "He can't hear or see us anymore because his soul and spirit are in heaven with Jesus, and it's so wonderful there he doesn't want to come back."

Francis pondered her answer and looked even more bewildered.

"We'll see him again when we go to heaven. Peter doesn't hurt anymore. In fact, he is perfect now, and we will be too when we get to heaven."

Still, Francis seemed unsure. Angel moved closer to her little brother and gently lifted his face so she could look into his eyes. "Franny, do you believe that Jesus died on the cross for your sins? For *all* of your sins, past, present, and future?" Angel asked.

Francis stared straight ahead.

Angel continued, "Have you asked Jesus to come into your life to be your personal LORD and Savior and promised to walk with Him in obedience?"

Perplexed, Francis nodded. That is what they had all been taught.

"Franny, someday you will see Peter again in heaven."

Francis didn't yet fully comprehend what his big sister conveyed to him. He knew that Jesus was the only way to heaven, and he was just beginning to learn who Jesus really was. But Angel planted the seeds, and his avenue to learning about Him was gradually beginning to open. It was Peter's death that made him think more about eternity.

The memory of Peter's death stayed with Francis for years. One day, Betty saw Francis laying out his stuffed Ernie and Bert dolls in little homemade coffins that he made out of shoeboxes he had lined with cloth diapers, like real caskets with linings. He was playing "undertaker." Rather discomfited, Betty asked him what on earth he was doing.

"I'm burying my childhood" was Francis's innocent reply.

In Tragedy We Trust

What carried the Smiths through Peter's untimely death was their faith in the unseen Jesus. Both acknowledged that their faithful LORD orchestrated Francis and Angel's homecoming so they could see their brother that one last time.

"Jesus doesn't make mistakes, and He decided He wanted to bring Peter home with Him," Betty told her inquisitive young son. "We can't possibly begin to understand why He chooses to do things that far surpass our limited understanding, but we still have to trust that He has His reasons. No matter what the outcome is, He has a plan. Someday, we will know what His plan is."

Betty was still in the midst of her own terrible grieving for Peter when she made that statement to Francis. There is nothing more devastating in the world than for parents to bury their child, and in the Smiths' case, they had buried several, the born and not yet born. Each and every loss was just as heartbreaking and overwhelming as the last one. There was no other pain like it, yet Bob and Betty kept their focus on Jesus and trust in His wisdom for their future. Later on, their suffering would enable them to be a blessing and a witness to other families who suffered through what they had. Continuously, they acknowledged their countless blessings. No matter what their heartache, they leaned on His promise that He would never abandon or forsake them. They believed all along that God had a plan and that He was at work in their lives in all things no matter how the circumstances appeared through their eyes. The family often took great comfort in Proverbs 3:4: "Trust in the Lord with all thine heart, and lean not unto thine own understanding. In all thy ways acknowledge Him, and He shall direct thy paths."

***

In spite of the family's tears and sadness, the two months following Francis's jaw surgery passed quickly. Through it all, Francis quietly persevered, just as he always did, even while he endured a liquid diet delivered by a syringe through his wired jaws and breathing through his temporary tracheostomy. When it came time to travel back to St. Louis to have his jaws unwired under anesthesia, Bob took him and stayed by his bedside.

There would be several more trips back to St. Louis over the years to come. Eventually, Bob and Betty decided to break the trip down with an overnight stay along the way. Straight off Exit 82 on Interstate 70 in Illinois was a motel that had a beautiful pyramid-roofed family restaurant on the property. The staff became friends with the Smiths and reveled in being a part of Francis's journey and recovery.

Pancakes Immortalized

Upon waking from his last surgery, his mouth was unwired, and the tracheostomy was removed. And he had a new chin! When the doctors asked him what he wanted to eat, without hesitation, he said, "Pancakes!" As they are today, pancakes have always been his favorite breakfast. The next morning, the doctors and nurses and several staff gathered around his bed for this most monumental event. To their delight, Francis's breakfast tray was loaded with a tall stack of pancakes topped with a generous dollop of butter and lots and lots of syrup! Apparently, Francis suffered no discomfort at all in chewing for the first time in two months. Perhaps he was too ecstatic to notice as he chowed down the huge stack of pancakes. Not until he had cleaned his plate and taken his last bite did he stop eating. Exhausted, the knife and fork dropped from his hands and onto the bedspread.

Francis's first pancake breakfast later inspired a family friend and Bob's co-worker, Brenda Joy Tucker, to write a poem to keep the memory and legend of his love of pancakes alive. Betty was so impressed with the poem she submitted it, along with the details of how it came to be, to their local newspaper, *The Evening Star*, for publication. The paper carried it along with a short letter from Betty, under the title, *The Legend of the Pancake Kid*.

The Legend of the Pancake Kid

I have a little story
I think I should tell.
It's about a little boy
We all know so well.

We asked, "What do you want to eat,
When you get your wires out?"
"Pizza, hot dogs, popcorn?"
"No!" he said with a shout.
"I want pancakes," we heard him utter.
"With lots of syrup and loads of butter."

And then came Wednesday,
Our faces were grim.
Could it be that our Francis
Finally got his new chin?
As the doctors worked,
We silently prayed.
Francis wasn't worried,
Not even afraid.

"It worked," said the doctor.
"It's a beautiful chin."
Francis looked up at us,
With a big silly grin.

He said, "It's time for the pancakes,"
As he jumped to his feet.
"Tomorrow," said the doctor,
"All you can eat."
The big day came.
He woke with a smile.
He would get his pancakes,
In just a little while.
In they came, piled really high.
Francis thought they would reach the sky.
He ate and ate 'til his stomach popped,
He put down his fork and let his arms drop.
"I've had enough.
My stomach is sore. Wait 'til tomorrow,
And I'll have some more."

There's a moral to this little story:
Believe in GOD to the end.
The Pancake Kid did,
And he got a brand-new chin...
                                    —Brenda Joy Tucker, 1982

Moving Forward

Due to his surgeries and the death of his brother, Francis was one month late returning to J. E. Ober Elementary School for first grade. His fondest memories of his elementary school years were his love for the extra-curricular classes in art, music, library time, and film time. It was the arts and his art teacher, Mr. Endress, who truly impressed him.

Betty admired her son's artwork that was spread across the dining room table, and she was quite amazed. Her youngest son delighted in drawing skyscrapers, airplanes, cities, Martian flying saucers, and various other subjects. What amazed her the most was his eye for detail and accu-racy. The Boeing 747 appeared to be his favorite subject, mostly because his dream from very early on was to fly in one. In fact, he was quite adamant that someday he was going to be a missionary, one who would "travel great dis-tances on a 747!" His depictions were amazingly accurate. As a "budding architect," he loved to "design" high-rise apartment buildings in cities. As a devoted science fiction fan, he loved to draw giant flying saucers landing on earth and unloading Martians. The books he loved to check out at the library supported his interest in airplanes, UFOs, space, or buildings. His fertile imagination was proving to be limitless, sometimes much to his family's chagrin. He could get quite caught up in his imagination, sometimes to the point of it becoming his inward reality, a trait common in autism.

Around this time, Francis continued his speech therapy through the school's program. Now that his jaw was properly aligned, he was finally able to work on his problem sounds: b, p, and f.

True to his autistic tendencies, Francis kept to himself. Playing alone on the playground equipment was preferable to the rowdy ball games that other students were involved in, which was just as well considering how small and frail he was for his age. Classmates were mostly acquaintances as opposed to friendships. However, he did make friends easily with adults. This was about the time he began to experience teasing, which sadly was just a prelude to the outright bullying he would be forced to endure a few short years later.

The Smith household always seemed to be in a constant whirlwind of change. Some of the children were in middle school or high school. The twins Rob and Becky were just starting school at Faith Christian Academy, attached to Bible Baptist Church, in nearby Auburn. James, who struggled mightily with his impulsive behavior problems that stemmed from his drug addiction at birth, now attended New Horizons, a special Christian boarding school for troubled teens, in Marion. Christopher attended Garrett Junior-Senior High School.

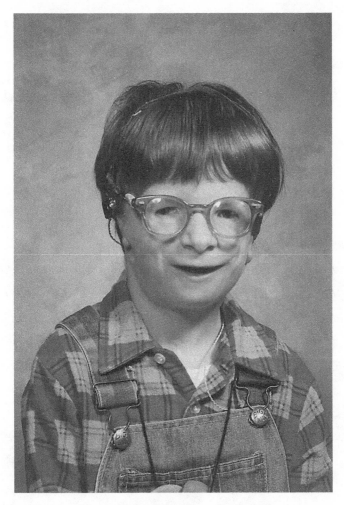

Francis, in the second grade.

Chapter 5

The Gospel Message of Jesus Christ

*Moreover, brethren, I declare unto you the gospel which
I preached unto you, which also ye have received, and
wherein ye stand; by which also ye are saved, if ye keep in
memory what I preached unto you, unless ye have believed
in vain. For I delivered unto you first of all that which I
also received, how that Christ died for our sins according
to the scriptures; And that He was buried, and that he
rose again the third day according to the scriptures.*

—1 Corinthians 1:1–4

*For God so loved the world,
He gave His only begotten Son,
that whosoever believeth in him
should not perish,
but have everlasting life.*

—John 3:16 (King James Version)

Christians are God's workmanship,
created for the purpose of good works.

—Charles Stanley

A New House of Worship

Bob had been raised in the Catholic church his entire life, a system of belief he devoutly followed and one that his wife and, later on, children embraced. Every evening, Bob faithfully led their children in evening prayer and devotion in the scripture-based *Our Daily Bread.* When he traveled, it was Betty who led the children. To the best of Bob and Betty's abilities, their children were raised to love and trust in their LORD.

But all was not well with their current church. This was the second church they attended as a family, and much to their ongoing disappointment, they were met by quite a bit of unease. Most people were polite, and a few even reached out to them, but over all, there was a sense of indignation and rejection. The way they were treated in the world was bad enough, but in their house of worship, it was intolerable.

And there is salvation in no one else; for there is no other name
under heaven that has been given among
men by which we must be saved.

—Acts 4:12

For God has not destined us for wrath,
but to obtain salvation through our Lord Jesus Christ,
who died for us
so that whether we are awake or asleep
we might live with him.

—1 Thessalonians 5:9–10

Born Again, the Angels Rejoice in Heaven

Jesus answered him,
"Truly, truly, I say to you,
unless one is born again
he cannot see the kingdom of God."

—John 3:3

Christianity starts with repentance.

—D. Martin Lloyd Jones

***

Salvation

Francis was raised in a God-loving, God-fearing (meaning *reverence* for God) family since he was two and a half years old. At the young age of six years old, he had faced the death of his beloved older brother, and with that experience came the ensuing questions about eternal life. Now, at nine years old, he had weathered a significant change in churches, hence, a new style of worship and subsequently a belief that was now Bible centered and not at all religious. His soul and spirit were constantly fed, and now he sought answers to the bigger questions.

Francis already had a basic childlike faith in Christ, and he understood that he was a sinner who was in need of a savior. He grasped Jesus's willing, obedient, sacrificial death on the cross for his sins that resulted in the *free* gift of salvation. Francis loved the verses in the Bible that somehow spoke personally to him. One verse that emphatically states the meaning of true salvation is a verse he memorized, Ephesians 2:8–9: "For by GRACE you are saved through FAITH; and not of yourselves: it is a GIFT of God: Not of works, lest any man should boast."

Through the steadfast nightly biblical teachings of his parents and now through the teachings of Sunday school, pastor, and church, Francis understood what biblical salvation and biblical baptism truly was. Baptism was instituted by Jesus Christ Himself, and it is a command, not a suggestion. Matthew 28:19–20: "Go and make disciples of all nations, baptizing them in the name of the Father and the Son and of the Holy Spirit, and teaching them to obey everything I have commanded you. And surely I am with you always, to the very end of the age." It is through baptism that a person is admitted into the fellowship of the church, meaning, the body of Christ.

In the Catholic church, Francis was sprinkled as an infant, yet infant baptism cannot be found anywhere in Scripture. The Bible's New Testament teaches that only believers who consciously and willingly place their faith and trust in Christ are baptized as a public testimony of their faith and identification with Him. An infant or very young child cannot possibly place his or her faith in Christ or make a conscious decision to obey Christ. How does pouring or sprinkling illustrate the death, burial, and resurrection of Jesus Christ? After all, Jesus Himself had been baptized at the age of thirty by John the Baptist in the Jordan River. Jesus was never sprinkled as a baby. Baptism, the Bible teaches, is an act of obedience. It is a public proclamation of faith after one is genuinely saved and born again.

Nor does baptism have anything to do with salvation. "Francis," Pastor Smith made clear, "baptism has nothing to do with your salvation. If you are genuinely saved and you die in a car crash on the way to get baptized, you are still going to heaven." Being "born again," Pastor Smith explained, was a spiritual rebirth where one aligns oneself with the one true God of the Bible and willingly eschews the ways of the world. In other words, it is when one agrees to follow the commands and ways of Jesus because they love and trust in Him, and they want their life to reflect that.

Finally, Francis was able to grasp what Pastor Smith was teaching him. Openly, he declared himself a sinner and admitted that the blood of Jesus washed away his sins on the cross, and the result was the free gift of salvation for all who believed in the gospel message. Before long, Francis felt ready to publicly profess his beliefs to his family and friends. The next step was baptism.

Biblical Baptism

Betty, who was raised solely on the Bible by her mother, never knew anything about man-inspired religion or the human tampered-with claims of one particular Christian denomination over another. Their faith was based solely on scriptures and nothing else, and that's what they lived by. Now that she and Bob and the children were worshipping in a Bible-preaching, Bible-teaching local church, the subject and importance of biblical baptism, in the name of the Father, Son, and Holy Spirit, was stirring her heart. Betty's desire was to be biblically baptized and publicly state her faith and commitment to obedience and discipleship in Christ along with her son, Francis. Together, mother and son were counseled by Pastor Smith to prepare them for their baptism.

Jesus began His public ministry at thirty-years old when he was baptized by John the Baptist which marked the beginning of his public ministry. Jesus was sinless, so why was He baptized? By doing so, He demonstrated that He was the Messiah, John 1:29: "the Lamb of God who takes away the sins of the world." His baptism was a sign of this great truth, and it was confirmed by God the Father Himself when Jesus came out of the water by declaring Matthew 3:17: "This is my Son, whom I love; with Him I am well pleased."

There was only one obstacle. Francis was desperately afraid of the water. Having spent most of his early childhood with a trach, whenever water was splashed on it, he was overcome by the terrible sensations of choking and drowning.

Biblical baptism by total immersion is a reenactment of the symbolic recreation of Christ's death, burial, and resurrection, meaning Francis would have to be tipped over onto his back and completely immersed into the water before rising out of the water again. Betty was deeply concerned about her son's hydrophobia and point-blank asked him if being baptized was what he really wanted. Without any hesitation, his answer was yes. Through collective prayer, Francis was able to overcome his fear of water long enough to be baptized.

"Bathing was always very difficult for Francis. During the years he had the tracheostomy, he was afraid of getting it wet. I was not concerned about him wanting to be baptized though. He wanted that so much," reminisced Betty.

One Sunday evening at church, Pastor Smith baptized both Betty and Francis, who was now ten, one right after the other. During the process of baptism, the congregation sang the slow reverent hymn "Where He Leads Me." Upon rising out of the water, they were received into their local church membership and into the body of Christ.

> *"We were all baptized by one Spirit so as to form*
> *one body—whether Jews or Gentiles, slave or free,*
> *and we were all given one Spirit to drink."*
>
> 1 Corinthians 12:13

*Having been buried with him in baptism, in which
you were also raised with him through your faith in the
working of God, who raised him from the dead.*
—Colossians 2:12

*For all of you who were baptized into Christ
have clothed yourselves with Christ.*
—Galatians 3:27

Chapter 6

The Story of Ruth
Spring 1983

Then Naomi her mother-in-law said to her,
"My daughter,
should I not seek rest for you,
that it may be well with you."

—Ruth 3:1

Where Have All the Children Gone?

By now, nearly all the older Smith children were enjoy-ing their independence, and some of them no longer lived at home. More often than not, Francis found himself in the playroom alone.

"All of our children were encouraged to be as inde-pendent as humanly possible," remembered Betty. Every step, each of their challenged children took toward having a life of their own and having the ability to function inde-pendently was met with complete gratitude from Bob and

Betty who gave all the glory to God for orchestrating their successes. The children either went to work as quickly as they were able, or they went off to college, and several of them did both.

"Becky worked as a carryout grocer in Auburn. Rob went on to college at Indiana Wesleyan University in Marion, Indiana. While Rob was still in high school, he had volunteered at the local veterinarian's office in town. He loved animals."

All the children adored animals, and there were plenty of them in the Smith household. The animals were of tremendous importance in teaching the children to love and responsibly care for something that depended on them. Early on when Edwin was still unable to connect emotionally with any of them, he became very attached to their Siamese cat. In fact, when she was pregnant and gave birth, he played delivery room nurse. When it came time to find homes for the kittens, Betty couldn't sell them. "I was very particular about finding the right homes for them, and it had nothing to do with money." They did keep one kitten though that quickly became the recipient of Edwin's doting care.

It would suffice to say that the Smiths were not quite suffering from empty nest syndrome, but there was definitely a lull in the family.

A New Sister for Francis

Francis appeared unfazed by being alone so much, but Betty and Bob knew it was not ideal for him. Neither of them sought to bring in another child, but the LORD thought differently.

In late spring, 1983, Francis was introduced to his new sister, Delana, who was known as Dee Dee, and she was three years old. Two years prior when she was barely one year old, she contracted a rare form of meningococcal meningitis. When she first became ill, her mother ignored her. Only after her conditions severely worsened did her grandmother and older sister rush her to the emergency room. By then, it was too late. Her fever had reached one hundred five degrees, and most of the skin on her body was either burned or infected. Gangrene resulted, necessitating the amputation of both of her legs above the knees along with several fingers from one hand. Even her nose was gone, and in its place was a gaping hole. Skin grafts covered her entire body. Inside the walls of Riley Hospital, Dee Dee was fighting for her life.

Immediately, Dee Dee was removed from her mother's custody. When Dee Dee's plight was brought to the attention of the Smiths, they did not hesitate for a moment to bring her into their family. When she arrived at the Smith home, all her meager belongings were carried inside a trash bag.

Betty was asked to work with Dee Dee's mother in order to help her cope with her daughter's challenges. "But her mother was not willing to work toward those goals," remembered Betty. However, sometime during that year, her mother did try to gain her back through the court system. There was a court hearing, and both Bob and Betty were fully expecting the court to place Dee Dee back with her mother, but much to their surprise, the judge thought otherwise. The bottom line was her mother was deemed negligent and unable to care for her. Since Dee Dee was doing so well with the Smiths, the judge decided that the Smith home was where she belonged. Betty and Bob could not have been happier.

As with all the Smith children, the first thing on their agenda was to find a more suitable family name for their newest daughter and sibling. During their nightly reading of *Our Daily Bread*, those who were still present in the house gathered quietly around the old round table as Bob opened the family Bible. In no time at all, "Ruth" was chosen as Dee Dee's new name. Not only was the story of Ruth and Naomi one of their family's favorites, but Ruth was also Betty's mother's name.

Almost immediately, Betty and Bob and his faithful insurance saw to it that Ruth received a Jobst Suit, a special suit for burn victims that was designed and made from knitted compression material that uses pressure to help burned skin (mostly covered with skin grafts) heal. Even her head was covered in a Jobst mask with holes for the eyes, nose, mouth, and ears. Much to the chagrin to the powers that be, Betty took it upon herself to cut out little holes in the headpiece that would allow her to wear pigtails. Boy, did she hear about that!

Promptly, and much to Ruth's delight, Betty set out to sew up a whole new wardrobe to accommodate her new daughter's challenges. First was a flowered-print sundress with matching bloomers, complete with a sunbonnet. Ruth was thrilled. Due to the skin grafts, she couldn't risk getting sunburned, so the new clothes were practical and protective as well as feminine and pretty.

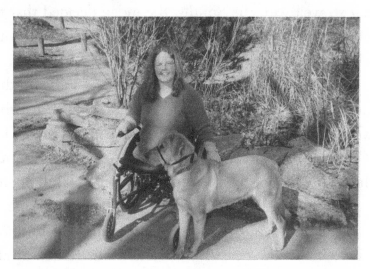

Ruth and her faithful companion, Bayleigh

After Ruth became a member of the Smith family, she endured the first of her many reconstructive surgeries. Never once did she complain. No one in the family was the least bit fazed by what she faced, especially Francis who had already experienced his own numerous surgeries and still had many more to come in his own future.

Fairly early into her rehabilitation, Ruth received her first pair of realistic-looking wooden artificial legs at an artificial limb clinic in Fort Wayne. Bob and Betty had been introduced to the man who made the artificial legs by hand. They were awkward and heavy and quite unwieldy, but out of sheer determination, a trait that Ruth showed very early in life, she somehow managed. At first, all she could do was stand on them. Ruth's dream was to wear a pair of little black patent-leather shoes that were all the rage back then, so Betty saw to it that she got them, and once they were strapped on, she was inspired to learn to walk on her new legs. Betty got her a pair of Canadian-style crutches—the kind that strap around the arm, and off she went. *Crutch, step…crutch, step…*What a marvelous sound!

An Immediate Bond

For all his life with the Smiths, Francis's strongest connection had always been with his big sister, Angel. Angel was twenty-two years old by now and was living her own life. She was married, and she and her husband were beginning a family of their own. Gradually, Francis's connection to his older sister began to lessen. Thankfully, his bond with Ruth was as immediate as it was strong. Ruth had a very strong competitive spirit, and the two soon developed a whopping case of sibling rivalry that only served to make them stronger together. They both shared a common trait; they were extremely smart. Ruth loved to play with her dolls (which, over the years, Francis loved to "operate" on, much to her horror) and cook on a toy kitchen set the nurses at Riley Hospital had given her, which was a prelude to her own real cooking skills that she later on developed. Much to the chagrin of her new family, she also liked to be waited on hand and foot, and she loved to order her big brother around. Betty didn't waste any time telling her that if she wanted to get ahead in this world, she had better start doing things on her own, which Francis wholeheartedly agreed. The whole family pitched in to help her gain independence and confidence in all areas of her life. Soon, the lessons sank in and served her well later on in her life.

***

Once Ruth mastered the use of her legs, it was clear that she wanted to go out into the world and do what other young girls her age were doing. Eagerly, her biggest desire was to learn to ride a tricycle. When word reached the physical therapy department at Riley Hospital, the staff rigged something up for her so she could have a trike to ride.

"Later on, we received a catalog from Switzerland that had a very special trike that was operated with your hands, but oh! It was so expensive," recalled Betty.

Unbeknown to Betty, a good friend of hers whose daughter went to school with Ruth and who was also a pastor's wife at another church put together a fund-raiser at her church to raise the money for the trike. One day, the trike from the catalog landed on their doorstep. It was a complete surprise, and she was thrilled. Ruth had the trike for years, and when she was too big to ride it anymore, she passed her prized possession on to another little girl.

Ruth the adventurer.

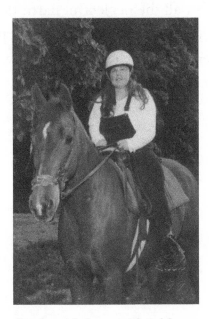

Ruth with her artificial legs.

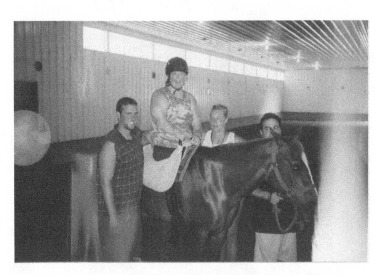

Ruth eventually decided to forego her artificial
legs and depend solely on her wheelchair.

Ruth would endure her own rocky journey to believing in Christ after all the neglectful harm that was done to her. Through the same steady guidance her parents gave to all their children, she now sees that God was with her all along. The outcome proves that.

Book 3

My soul clings to You:
Your right hand upholds me.

—Psalm 63:8

Chapter 1

Back to Francis
1983–1984

Craniofacial Mishaps

Francis soon was faced with another facial surgery to reconstruct his missing cheekbones and lower eye socket rims and to build his outer ears that would entail rib grafts, wires, and screws. As a bonus, Dr. Marsh and his team were also going to make fake earlobes from pelvic bone and skin grafts.

However, the first part of these surgeries almost ended in crisis. During the building of his right eye socket, a nerve was damaged, and over a period of six or so months, Francis became permanently blind in that one eye. Much to the astonishment of his doctors and family, who were all extremely upset about it, he remained nonchalant about the incident. Bob and Betty were only glad that the other eye could be saved. Eye doctors tried patching the left eye in order to force the right eye to learn to see again, but that was unsuccessful. Subsequently, Francis wore prescription glasses for a year, again without success. Never one to complain about such things, he took what most would consider a setback in stride and went about his business as if nothing had happened. After all, he still had one eye from which he could see. Now he was missing the ability to perceive depth, and even that didn't seem to perturb him either.

The surgery that followed also had an unhappy outcome. Francis was to be given cheek implants in order to have greater facial structure. Shortly after his new cheekbones were implanted, Betty happened to pass by Francis's room. She stopped in her tracks. Francis was preening in front of his mirror. "Oh, you handsome boy you," he was saying. He was so proud of his new face Betty could only laugh. A short while later though, one of the implants became infected, requiring that both cheek implants be removed. Again, Betty was left bereft by this setback, but Francis shrugged it off. He still had two new ears to admire with his one good eye, and to him, he was wonderfully made!

"Don't worry, Mom. I'm alive," he stoically said. Such was the positive attitude of Francis Joel Smith.

Camping: The Smith Family Tradition

The Smiths were a large happy family, and by choice, they did everything they possibly could do, together.

Before Betty married Bob, she had introduced him to camping, something she had enjoyed all the way back to her childhood. So, from the very beginning of their marriage, camping became a family tradition.

For the first few years after Francis arrived, Bob and Betty held off on camping because of Francis's serious medical condition, his early surgeries, and the necessity of feeding him through tubes.

Camping at Chain O'Lakes, 1983.

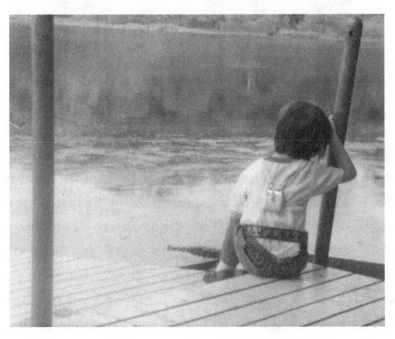

Francis sitting on the dock.

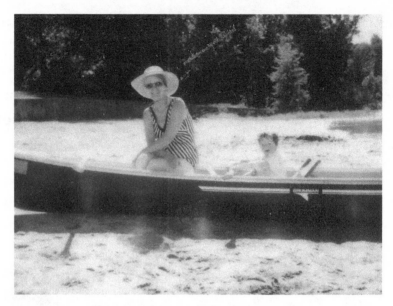

Betty and Francis in their canoe.

From the summer of 1983, Chain O'Lakes State Park became the Smith family's traditional summer camping spot; it provided an ideal campground with handicap-accessible asphalt sites that they always used. They enjoyed hiking and visiting the nature center that was housed in an old one-room schoolhouse converted for that purpose. Betty, especially, loved the beach at Sand Lake, and they all loved swimming. By the second summer, Bob and Betty purchased a beautiful green canoe with paddles and life jackets so they could enjoy paddling the network of channels connecting most of the lakes at Chain O'Lakes. Without fail, however, serious rain showers tagged along, year after year. Francis was not the least bit enamored by the rain, but for the sake of family tradition, he willed himself to accept it as an uninvited but tolerated guest during their camping fun. The family camping trips are among his favorite memories of being a member of the Smith family. Francis, however, never did get over his fear of water, so he always refused to go swimming. Playing in the sand though was something he dearly loved, along with canoeing. Eventually, he even learned to paddle on his own. Hiking became a lifelong habit that came to serve him well during his later adventures.

A Most Surprising Little Maestro

In the spring of 1984, Bob and Betty got the surprise of their lives; Francis began playing the piano. The Smiths were a very musical household. Angel's biological parents were music professors, so it was only logical that she would have inherited their talent. Most of the others had learned to play the piano, guitar, and other instruments, so these instruments were often lying around and accessible. It was only natural that Francis would play around with these instruments and experiment with them. The thought of him actually learning to play these instruments was an entirely different matter. Bob and Betty never really gave it any thought.

One Sunday morning, the Sunday school teacher approached Bob and Betty and asked if they would mind if Francis played the doxology for class on the piano. At first, they both thought the teacher was joking. After all, Francis had never had any formal music training. Besides, for all intents and purposes, he was deaf. Somehow, the teacher managed to convince them that their son really was quite capable. "So could he please?" They both gave their consent, but still, they didn't quite believe it.

Then they heard him play. His ear for pitch, tone, and beat was flawless! Considering Francis was only able to hear through vibration, this completely baffled his family.

Needless to say, in very short order, Francis was signed up for piano lessons. Mrs. Geneva Nissly, an older white-haired lady who lived across town and who taught a few of the other Smith children, acquired him as her latest pupil. Starting with the basics, she taught him how to read and play music. Miraculously, he caught on rapidly, which was no small feat for someone who didn't even have a pair of ears. The two became very close, and they continued to work together for several years until she and her husband relocated to Florida. It was through her that he learned to express himself beautifully through music, something Francis is deeply indebted to her. After Mrs. Nissly and her husband retired to Florida, Betty searched for another piano teacher. They got in touch with the pianist at church, Mrs. Kelsey, who also happened to be a piano teacher. Originally, it was thought that Mrs. Kelsey would be too demanding a teacher for Francis with all his challenges, but they soon discovered that she actually was the best teacher for him. A trained classical pianist, Mrs. Kelsey proved very patient while working with Francis. Under her tutelage, he built an even more solid classical background. The two of them formed a strong bond that lasted well into his high school years.

An Untapped World of Music

It wasn't long before Francis's accomplishment on the piano led him to branch out into other musical areas. Several of his siblings were also musically inclined, and finding various instruments lying around the house was a common sight. As inquisitive as he was, he didn't hesitate to pick up the instruments and play with them. Before long, he was holding his own among his musically talented brothers and sisters in filling the Smith household with marvelous music on a near daily basis. A 1914 Hobart M. Cable upright piano was acquired, and for his musical debut, he played "Joy to the World" for their family and friends' Christmas gathering. Not long afterward, he even learned to play the violin that later on became his second favorite instrument to play. Not the least bit shy from that point on, he became a common musical presence in their church and at other social gatherings through the years. This was just one more of the many miraculous gifts that were, and would continue to be, given to him in the future.

Steadfast in the LORD (1984)

Nothing filled Bob's and Betty's hearts with greater joy than watching their children grow in faith and overcome their individual challenges, step-by-step, as they learned to navigate their most difficult challenges. To them, every step their children took was nothing less than miraculous.

One thing Bob and Betty refused to tolerate from any of their children was to hear them say, "I can't." Or to give in to self-pity or to succumb to the attitudes of others who simply could not see beyond their own narrow vision of what was "normal." Constant prayer and diligent faith in the LORD is what gave them that strength.

***

Although by now the older children were well on their way, Francis—and now Ruth—were still facing multiple surgeries that were necessary in order to give them what they needed to keep them moving forward. All along, Bob and Betty believed that God had very special plans for their children, and their job was to see that they achieved them.

With a sense of relief, 1984 was anticipated to be a much easier year for Francis in terms of surgeries. Having three crowns put on three different teeth along with having dental impressions for a planned future palate speech appliance was fairly simple by comparison to the seriousness of several of his earlier surgeries. Francis was scheduled for anesthesia for the crowns and speech appliance that would be delivered through a rather tricky nasal-tracheal intubation.

Unexpectedly, Francis repeatedly kept waking up during the procedure, and he had to be put back under again and again, which was very wearing for all concerned. The end result was he ended up having to stay overnight at Riley Hospital. Not to mention, there was still another long drive back to St. Louis that fall for the third stage of Francis's earlobe reconstruction. For the Smiths, all of this was just another day's work in their lives, and they took it all in stride, with the LORD by their side.

An Incredible New Family Adventure

As Francis's multiple craniofacial surgeries were proving to be successful, more opportunities began to unfold. Sometime during that spring, the doctors and staff at Riley Hospital informed Bob and Betty of two special summer camps for children with serious speech disorders. Ball State University in Muncie, where Susie had attended, offered a program they were already familiar with. Now there was another program being offered by the University of Michigan. They looked deeply into both programs, comparing the advantages versus the disadvantages along with the costs.

After a great deal of soul-searching and prayer, Bob and Betty were led to the University of Michigan's program, believing that this one would best meet their son's needs. It was an intensive speech therapy program offered in a summer camp setting for a six-week session. The program incorporated opportunities for socialization and recreation while focusing intently on correcting serious speech problems. Since Francis was socially withdrawn and still quite noncommunicative, this was the primary reason this camp was chosen over the other.

That spring, Bob and Betty submitted Francis's application for the summer session of 1984, from July 1 through mid-August, a full six weeks. However, there was a major obstacle that had to be faced. The cost of the camp was prohibitive—it was nearly two thousand dollars. (This would amount to nearly ten thousand dollars by today's standards.) Bob's insurance would not cover this, so where on earth would they get the money?

Bob and Betty and the family prayed together for a financial miracle that would allow Francis to have the opportunity he so badly needed. Bob diligently began to approach various charitable organizations in hopes of getting the funds, but for one reason or another, he was turned down by all of them. There wasn't much time before the full amount was due, and through their eyes, the situation looked hopeless. Bob repeatedly reminded his family, "Keep your eyes on the LORD, not the situation."

***

Since the camp was a major distance away, the Smiths decided that this time would be turned into a family summertime adventure. Bob managed to take some vacation time in order to pack up the entire family—kids, dogs, cats, and all—for a weeklong camping trip so they could all remain close to Francis for his first week at camp if the need should arise.

Getting Francis ready was a major ordeal all by itself. Packing for six weeks was not easy especially for someone with special needs. Clothing, toiletries, glasses, hearing aids, and batteries would all be needed. And last but not least, a place had to be made for Francis's beloved companion, Curious George. His army canvas duffle bag was packed to the hilt. The rest of the family had to pack too, not to mention the Smiths were even bringing their cats! The big brown Buick station wagon and the Apache fold-down trailer were packed to the gills.

The drive from Garrett in northeast Indiana to the far northwest corner of Michigan took an entire day. They arrived late at night, exhausted, at a campground called Whispering Pines near Grand Traverse Bay. In no time at all, they set up their trailer and the Add-A-Room and went to bed in their sleeping bags.

On the morning of the big day, the Smiths awoke early to a magnificent sunny summer morning. Their camp-site was carpeted with pine needles that shimmered with morning dew. After breakfast, they gathered into the sta-tion wagon for a rather lengthy drive to Shady Trails Camp, located a few miles south of the small city of Northport on Grand Traverse Bay.

Immediately off the highway was the camp entrance. They were greeted by the gorgeous red, green, and other rustic-colored log cabins that were strung together by roads and trails in the midst of a lush woods setting, overlook-ing the beautiful sandy beach used for swimming along the shore of Grand Traverse Bay. Other buildings were art-fully dispersed among the cabins. The setting was so allur-ing everyone had to take in a deep breath. After getting Francis checked in, they were shown to the cabin named Park Avenue, which was painted red. Like the others, it appeared small on the outside, but once inside, it was actually quite spacious.

There were four bunk rooms: three for campers and one for the cabin counselors, and each bunk room slept four to six boys. Toward the rear of the cabin was a large communal bathroom. Dominating the cabin was the main room, complete with a massive stone fireplace. Chairs and tables gave the room a comfortable rustic look. At night, in front of the crackling fire, the counselors loved to tell scary ghost stories, complete with sound effects. As soon as Francis was shown his room, Bob and Betty helped him unpack and get his belongings put away in closets and dresser drawers. Curious George even got settled in. He got his own special bed in the bottom bed of Francis's bunk.

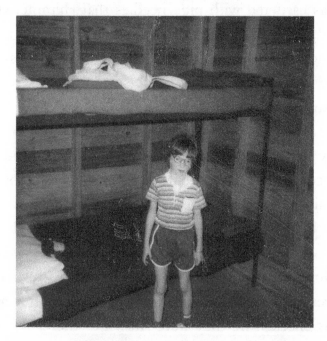

Francis by his bunk at camp.

Francis on His Own

After Francis was unpacked, Bob and Betty said their goodbyes then retreated to their own campground. They wanted their son to acclimate to his new surroundings as quickly as possible and on his own. They need not have worried, for he settled in without any problems.

That first day, the campers and counselors participated in icebreaker games and activities in order to get to know one another. Within hours, Francis had made friends with his two cabin counselors, Mr. McAllister and Mr. Jackson. He also got to know a few of his several cabinmates by name.

The structure and routine for the next six weeks was quickly established. Rise and shine was at seven o'clock sharp in the morning. Breakfast, lunch, and dinner were served family style at the same time every day in the beautiful modern wooden lodge-style dining hall with huge plate glass windows that overlooked the bay. Each cabin group ate meals at a large harvest-style dining table, and to Francis's recollection, their home-style meals were almost as good as his mom's cooking! It was here that he acquired his taste for raisin bran cereal, which was his breakfast staple for many years.

The camp activities were counselor led and designed to foster communication and interaction between campers. A large variety of games were constantly played along with the traditional camping activities such as hiking, swimming, singing, and canoeing. The campers learned the buddy system and employed it wherever they went but especially when they were near water. Swimming seemed to be a favorite for most of the campers. Francis gravitated mostly toward arts and crafts where he learned drawing, rock polishing, and other artistic activities. Once a week, they visited the camp's small library in the speech therapy building.

One of the more unusual activities was a hole-digging contest that took place in a clearing outside Francis's cabin. He once bragged that he could dig a hole all the way to the earth's core.

Amazing Breakthroughs

Camp activities were not all about play. They were designed for learning and responsibility as well. The campers were all assigned daily individual and group chores to teach them responsibility in working together to help run the camp. Francis relished his job as the cabin mail delivery boy.

While it was "safe" to learn, grow, and thrive among themselves, the outside world was where they would eventually have to learn to live, and that was far more daunting. Once or twice a week, the campers were taken on "out trips." Loaded into a fleet of dark blue Dodge passenger vans, the campers were driven into Northport, a short drive up the highway, or to a local beach or some other spot. This is where they got to practice their new speech and communication skills in public. One adventure Francis enjoyed the most was going inside a store to buy something. There he was expected to communicate with his new speech sounds and skills, and the reaction and attention he got was always glowing. What he especially loved was buying toy airplanes and helicopters from the variety stores, so boy, oh, boy, he learned very quickly to communicate well when it came to getting something he really wanted. Most of his model planes he bought unhappily disappeared over the years. Usually, they got caught up in a tree or crashed over the back fence, but one of his most special planes survived and remains with him to this day. It is a replica of a Cessna floatplane of the type used in Alaska. Made from blue plastic, it is a little over a foot long, complete with pontoons that had little wheels under them. Inside its molded plastic fuselage, it even had seats. No wonder, he fell in love with it at first sight. Back then, it only cost a dollar, but today, it remains a priceless and prized relic.

An avid rock collector, Francis purchased a Michigan Petoskey stone from a rock shop and then polished it himself. That stone remained a treasured possession for years.

One of Francis's fondest camp memories is when the campers slept outdoors at night, something they were allowed to do from time to time. Fortunately, there were no mosquitoes around, so it was quite a magical adventure to sleep in the open air with the stars twinkling above. The next morning, he woke up early and sat up, waiting for the great big orange fireball to inch its way over the horizon. He watched in wonder as the morning light gave life to his surroundings long before the others began to awaken.

This is one memory that stands out above so many other wonderful memories of his time spent at camp.

Fishing, Francis style, remains one of his mother's favorite tales. He caught his first fish in the big lake, but instead of having it for dinner, he was allowed to keep it as a pet. He named it George, after his beloved stuffed Curious George. Every day, he cared responsibly for George the Fish, talking to it and feeding it, making sure its water was fresh. He was very proud of it and the care he provided for it. At the end of camp, Francis returned his pet fish back to his lake home. The fish, for many reasons, was most likely hugely relieved.

Camp was full of great fun activities, but the real business at hand was to provide an intense individual speech therapy program for the kids. Every weekday, speech therapy was a part of the program. Francis was assigned Ms. McLain, who was definitely attractive. Every day, they met in the speech building. The speech offices were set up practically the same as the ones he was used to at Riley Hospital. With word cards and special picture flipcharts, Ms. McLain thoroughly worked with him on his problem sounds: b and p. He repeated those target sounds over and over, slowly beginning to improve by closing his lips and letting the sounds "pop" from his mouth through pursed lips. He worked both independently as well as in group sessions with Ms. McLain. It was work, but it was also fun and a great bonding experience for the kids, not to mention he was progressing in leaps and bounds. Francis's progress was dutifully charted by Ms. McLain every weekday. It was encouraging for Francis to see his progress every day from the beginning through the end of camp. As the summer progressed, each cabin was given the opportunity to showcase newly learned speech skills by designing and performing a cabin play in front of the entire camp community. Not exactly for the fainthearted! Each weekend, a different cabin staged its own uniquely, creatively designed play.

As much as Francis loved camp, like most of the others, he could barely contain himself when the mail arrived. This was the longest time away from his family he had ever spent, and the only way he could keep up and keep them informed of his endeavors was to write letters. Betty and Bob's letters were filled with how things were going at home. In their first letter, they described a violent rainstorm they experienced at Whispering Pines, a one-and-the-same storm the speech camp was experiencing several miles away. Only, he was in a cabin. They were in a trailer, and the Add-A-Room collapsed with everyone in it! Everything, including all of them, was drenched, and to this day, that tale is still told. The next week's letter contained a clipping of the newspaper article from *The Evening Star* telling of the Smiths' struggles to send their son to this very special camp. Francis, in turn, wrote about his camp adventures and updates on his speech progress. The fish story, however, remains one of their favorites.

As mid-July approached, the camp prepared for parents' visitation day. All the parents and guardians of the campers descended upon the camp to visit with their campers and to see how they were doing. This time, Bob and

Betty drove all night from their home in Garrett, Indiana, and straight through to Michigan without the benefit of a break. Arriving midday and without any sleep, they managed to spend a large portion of the day with Francis, touring his cabin and meeting his fellow campers and counselors before collapsing from exhaustion. Together, the next day, they drove to Northport where they spent several hours watching Francis practice his new skills. They ate at a quaint little ice cream parlor and spent some time sitting on the town pier, all the while talking and watching the sailboats on Grand Traverse Bay. Bob and Betty were amazed by how far their son had come and how much he was enjoying the camp. All too soon, their special day was over, and Francis stood and waved goodbye as the brown Buick station wagon disappeared from camp and back onto the highway.

From that point on, the camp days flew by at warp speed and were rapidly nearing an end. Before Francis knew it, the campers were packing up and getting ready to go home. There was no doubt that the amazing breakthrough Francis achieved in just a few short weeks would have taken months, or possibly even years, had he not been able to attend this outstanding specialized camp. Francis had mastered his most difficult obstacles. Again, the Smiths praised the LORD for providing their son with such a marvelous experience and the sorority that sponsored him.

During the last couple of weeks, the camp put on nightly dances after dinner. There were many closing activities during the last week, but the most anticipated was awards night. Each of the campers received a unique award for an interesting characteristic they showed or for something special they achieved. Francis received his award for being the most "curious" camper of all! He was constantly asking the most questions.

The last day of camp was upon them before they even knew it. Once again, parents and guardians converged on the camp, only this time it was to take their little campers home. It was a bittersweet moment for Francis when the brown Buick arrived and got parked. It was a day of final conferences with counselors and speech therapists, packing up, eating, and saying their last goodbyes. Bob and Betty were helping Francis pack his large army canvas bag into the station wagon when it was discovered that Curious George was missing. Francis ran back inside his cabin to find him, but his most treasured stuffed companion couldn't be found anywhere. Despondent, Betty and Bob and a few counselors and campers searched high and low for Curious George. Finally, they had to accept that he was gone. Francis was heartbroken, as was just about everyone else. No one ever knew what really happened. It is only a guess that Curious George was now in someone else's possession, probably not living the good life he had enjoyed with his first owner. That was the last time Francis ever saw his beloved Curious George, and he was absolutely heartbroken.

***

There was one last task at hand. Francis, Bob, and Betty had to pull themselves together for their final session with Ms. McLain. She made an audio tape of their last session together so his parents, doctors, and future speech therapists could have an audio record of the progress in his speech over the camp session. He still has this tape that has preserved his high-pitched nine-year-old voice with his therapist encouraging him to repeat words like "bat" over and over again until he got it right. Sometimes, to this day, he pulls this tape out of his archives and listens to it, amazed at how far his voice has come to this day and what work still needs to be done.

Now it was time to go. Twice previously, Francis had stood and waved goodbye to the receding station wagon as his parents drove off to home after their visit with him. This time, he was inside the station wagon, waving goodbye to a receding Shady Trails Camp. He kept his nose pressed to the window until he had his last glance, a vision that is etched in his memory forever.

Francis didn't really want to leave. Besides bestowing him with some of his fondest childhood memories, the speech camp quite literally provided him with the gift of verbal communication. At the beginning of camp, he was basically nonverbal because his speech was so impaired he wasn't understood. By the end of camp, everyone was clearly amazed at how he had mastered the most difficult sounds in as few as six weeks. He learned to speak slowly and clearly so others could understand him. The camp also taught him to socialize with others, something he could never do before. He made friends not only with the adults and counselors but among his peers as well. That was a huge breakthrough for him.

The following year, in third grade, Francis was asked to write about his experiences at speech camp in a young authors' competition book, which he titled *Curious George Goes to Camp*. After he wrote it, Betty loaned it to the women of the sorority who had provided the funding for him to go to speech camp. The book has not been seen again since.

Chapter 2

God Is Good
1985

An Advocate for Francis

There was no question in Bob's and Betty's minds as to where they wanted Francis to attend school, and that was Faith Christian Academy where Becky was in her senior year there. Ruth began attending kindergarten at the same time as Francis began the fourth grade. Unfortunately, for the same reasons as before, they faced opposition again, this time from school administration and teachers. His physical hardships, speech and hearing impediments were frightening to others.

Thankfully, Francis was already in the church's primary Sunday school class, and he was doing quite well. Still, there was quite a bit of opposition from the administration and reluctance from a couple of concerned teachers that kept him from attending the school. Undeterred, Bob and Betty kept up their pursuit and their prayers on behalf of their son.

Sometime in the fall of 1985, their prayers were answered. Keith Wittebols, the fourth-grade teacher, became aware of their plight. He questioned the powers that be as to why Francis was not being accepted into the school, and from that point on, he too became a relentless advocate on his behalf. Before long, Francis became a student in Mr. Wittebols's fourth-grade class.

"I remember meeting Mr. Wittebols on the first day of class," Francis recalled. "He was a tall slender man with bushy light-brown hair and a mustache, who struck a commanding pose at the front of the classroom in his tweed coat and square-ended knit tie." His first impression didn't end there. Mr. Wittebols's special way with children was captivating. His no-nonsense way of teaching and his obvious love and enthusiasm for his students captured their full attention from the very beginning. Learning was fun! Instead of relying solely on flashcards and rote memorization, he incorporated games and other activities that brought their learning material to life. Instead of sitting at their desks soaking up their lessons, the children were learning by interacting and forming strong bonds with one another along the way.

It was in Mr. Wittebols's class that Francis developed his love of science. He was fascinated by the experiments and their outcomes, and he eventually began to "plan" to become a doctor.

Each morning began with Bible reading and a short lesson followed by prayer. The blessings didn't stop there. The school was growing, and at a parent-teacher meeting later that year, Mr. Wittebols lobbied for another teacher. Betty rose to the challenge, and she soon became a volunteer teacher for the next year. Betty taught alongside Mr. Wittebols in his now-combined fourth-and-fifth-grades classroom. By that time, Francis was in the fifth grade, but he was still with Mr. Wittebols. While Mr. Wittebols taught Francis and the other fifth graders, Betty taught the fourth graders. The new schedule was worked out so that Francis was never actually in her class. At the end of the year, Mr. Wittebols was named teacher of the year.

Learning Interrupted (1986)

After Christmas break, Francis did not immediately return to his fourth-grade class. Another trip to St. Louis was scheduled for him in order for his surgeon to fine-tune the outer ears that were previously built. This was not supposed to be a difficult surgery, but it did require that he be put under with anesthesia.

However, this time, administering anesthesia proved to be a far more challenging ordeal than they imagined. Francis woke up in the recovery room, feeling no pain. Neither was there a telltale bandage wrapped around his head. Perplexed, he wondered whether or not the surgery had even happened. It wasn't until he was back in his room with Bob that a nurse explained that the surgery had to be discontinued because the anesthesiologist was unable to put him completely under. He kept waking up during the multiple attempts to insert a breathing tube into his throat through his mouth, first with a regular laryngoscope (a tool with a lighted blade to help see the vocal cords and insert the breathing tube into the airway) and then with a fiberoptic scope (a long thin flexible tube with a fiberoptic light in it). His throat was, and is, very narrow and prone to blockage of the tongue, thus making it difficult to see his vocal cords with either instrument, let alone insert a breathing tube down it. The airway has to remain open during anesthesia by the breathing tube so the oxygen and anesthetic gases can flow into the lungs. Unable to secure his airway with a breathing tube, the surgeon reluctantly called a halt to his surgery and sent him back to recovery. From that point on, the doctors at St. Louis Children's Hospital and, subsequently, Riley Hospital had to come up with other ways to anesthetize him.

A Mother's Day to Remember

In almost no time at all, Mother's Day was upon them. To celebrate this momentous occasion, Bob made plans for a family outing to the Ponderosa Buffet Steakhouse in Auburn where Betty could be doted on and indulge in her favorite meal. All the children were there for this greatly anticipated family event. As usual, the Smiths didn't just walk into a restaurant unnoticed. The arrival of this eclectic family brought the usual nudges and stares while the family stood in full view while waiting for their table.

Betty looked absolutely radiant on her special day. She bought a new dress for this occasion, and Bob pinned her with a delicate corsage. No one was prouder of her family on that day than she was.

Francis, as always, ordered his special breakfast of pancakes and link sausage. Since Francis's first jaw surgery in 1982, there had been some slippage in the alignment of his jaw that was causing an increasing difficulty in chewing and swallowing, but surgery, it was decided, would be put off until a later date, a decision that later on resulted in a life-or-death catastrophe.

Halfway through the brunch, Francis choked on a sausage link. Wheezing desperately and grabbing his throat, he gasped for air. The sausage lodged in his esophagus, allowing him some but not much air. He began to turn blue. A waitress ran to call 911, and Bob threw his son over his knee and began beating him on his back in an attempt to dislodge the sausage. The restaurant was in chaos as frightened diners stopped eating and began to cry and pray. Betty and the children were frantic! Sirens announced the arrival of the ambulance. Without preamble, Francis was loaded into the ambulance with his father with him. Betty gathered the children and got them into the station wagon as quickly as humanly possible, considering some of their limitations. She drove like a maniac—pedal to the metal, as they say—no doubt breaking the law along the way. Frantic, she had no idea what to expect when she got to the emergency entrance where the ambulance sat empty in front of the door. There was no sign of Bob.

Betty was led immediately into her son's cubicle while the children were left in the waiting area. Bob had thought to call Pastor Smith who arrived with his wife who arrived nearly at the same time as Betty. They gathered in prayer around Francis's hospital bed while Francis gasped and gurgled. There was nothing the medical staff could do! Riley Hospital was alerted, and Francis was loaded into another ambulance. This time, Betty rode in the ambulance while Bob drove the car. Pastor Smith and his wife followed.

It is not a short distance to Indianapolis. Under normal driving circumstances, it was a two-and-a-half-hour drive. With sirens blaring, the ambulance was driven at breakneck speed on the freeway, over several sets of railroad tracks and into the city. Betty felt for certain they wouldn't survive their wild ride. Finally, they arrived at the emergency entrance where the doctor and nurses greeted the ambulance.

In no time, Francis was rushed into the emergency room (ER) cubicle where he was surrounded by the emergency medical team. Betty was right there beside him. In moments, Bob joined them. He must have had quite a time keeping up with the ambulance with a station wagon full of children—but he did. Betty was surprised that her husband hadn't been pulled over. She gave thanks to the LORD for keeping them all together.

Upon examination, Francis was completely fine and totally nonchalant despite all the excitement. After a collective huge sigh of relief, the doctor diagnosed the sausage had probably been dislodged when the ambulance hit the bumps of numerous railroad tracks they had crossed along the way. For whatever reason, Francis never mentioned it to anyone. He was probably enjoying the excitement of the wild ride with the sirens blaring. What kid wouldn't?

Betty thought to tell the children immediately who were all huddled in the waiting room, anxious and scared about their little brother's fate. Others were there too, waiting to learn about their loved ones who, for whatever reason, were also there on Mother's Day. What a sight their children must have been, with their challenges and different races, clinging to one another in deep reverent prayer. They attracted attention wherever they went, but praying together in the emergency room waiting area must have been something else.

Betty was a welcome sight to her children as she emerged from the emergency room with a huge smile on her face. The children ran to greet her, embracing her in a huge hug. Bob and the Smiths were right behind her. Right then and there, they gathered with the children, prayed, and gave thanks to the LORD for saving Francis from what could very well have been a serious tragedy. In a few moments, a nurse brought Francis out who, as usual, just stood there soaking up all the attention. Without a doubt, this was Betty's most memorable Mother's Day.

A Wake-up Call

There was no putting off Francis's lower jaw reconstruction surgery after that very, very close call. That summer, Francis was back in the St. Louis hospital for a lower jaw reconstruction that involved the splitting of the jaw on each side and repositioning it using special-shaped metal plates and screws to hold it in place. Once again, he would endure his jaws being wired tightly shut for six weeks with a hospitalization required for at least one week. Old pro that he was, Francis had no complaints about being back on his blenderized diet, which, quite frankly, he rather enjoyed. The family even went on a camping trip for a few days, and Betty brought along the blender. By now, she was the master of many special recipes that her son claimed were gourmet.

But this surgical journey was not without some true-to-Francis-style excitement. The trach that enabled him to breathe dislodged from his throat one night, requiring an emergency trip to Parkview Memorial Hospital ER. The hole had started to close, preventing the reinsertion of the tube. Somehow, Francis was able to breathe without it, so they let it be, and he was fine.

School Again—Not So Much Fun

Francis loved to learn, and he had looked forward to the new school year with great anticipation. Unfortunately, he was in for a rather rude surprise. Gone was his beloved Mr. Wittebols who had taught him in the fourth and fifth grades. Now in the sixth grade, he was faced with new teachers and new ways. Staying true to his love of music and his expanding expertise on various instruments, he signed up for band, meaning, drums were now a part of his instrument repertoire. Much to his family's chagrin, Francis practiced drums at home. At first, he enthusiastically embraced his new musical classes and caught on quickly to learning another new instrument, the xylophone. It didn't take much time though before his joy of music began to wane, for Francis's relationship with his band teacher began to sour. After the first year, his teacher began to demonstrate impatience with Francis that developed slowly, at first, but then quickly worsened. It wasn't just with him either. The instructor began to show a lack of tolerance toward all the children that made the class tense to the point of being nearly unbearable. For Francis, due to his heightened sensitivity toward situations, this had an extremely adverse effect. Increasingly, whenever a student made a wrong note during rehearsal, the band director would lash out and throw a baton or a stick at the student who made the error. Francis himself was the unwitting victim of this behavior many times over. Or worse, the bandleader would kick over the music stand, terrorizing all of them.

Francis never shared this with Betty. He kept his anxiety over the escalating situation to himself. One day, Francis had enough. In protest of the treatment he was receiving, he played hooky. Summoned to the bandleader's office, he experienced a chewing out that frightened him to death. Still, he remained silent about it. Again, he played hooky, only this time he failed to show up for the spring concert. Again, he was summoned to the office. He promptly quit band with no explanation to his parents.

While band had been a choice, chorus was not. It was a requirement for all elementary school students, and much to Francis's deep unhappiness, he didn't like being in choir any better than he had the band teacher. His love for music and his trust in his instructors diminished to the point he began to lose his interest in music. Since her son did not voice his unhappiness with the situation, Betty was perplexed by his growing distance in what was once his greatest pleasure. He still had wonderful relationships with his piano teachers, but from that point on, he had no desire to have anything to do with choir or band. At best, he went through the motions without experiencing any enjoyment.

Summer Vacation, Hospital Style

In the spring of 1987, Bob, Betty, and even Ruth accompanied Francis for the long trek to St. Louis for his all-day outpatient evaluation with Dr. Marsh. He was measured, weighed, poked, prodded; and his eyesight and hearing were tested. By the end of this trying long day, the craniofacial deformities team had written up a thorough multipage summary of his evaluation. Recommendations were written up for his future surgeries in the years ahead.

For most of the summer of 1987, Francis was hospitalized. Dr. Marsh felt it was time to remove the artificial palate mouthpiece Francis had been wearing since the failed first attempt to close the opening with his tongue flap and reattempt the tongue flap again. Once again, his mouth was wired shut, and he breathed through a trach. Remembering the near catastrophe of tearing his tongue flap down from his palate in his sleep in 1982, no chances were taken. He awoke from the surgery with stiff restraint splints wrapped around both his arms that tied him to the bed.

The next few weeks at home passed by uneventfully. Back in St. Louis, the surgery was deemed a success, and his arm splints were removed, and so was the mouthpiece that covered up the hole in his palate. However, years later, he did notice that the tongue flap had not completely covered the fistula, and it remains open to this day. This time, Francis was able to return to the new school year on time, unlike the delays other surgeries had imposed on him.

Accolades for Betty

Through the years, Bob and Betty had become role models for other adoptive parents of special needs children and were often singled out to speak to groups of prospective families and adoption agencies. It was, therefore, not the least bit surprising that Betty was honored with the prestigious mother of the year award from a midwestern parenting organization based in Chicago. Most exciting of all was Francis was invited to accompany his mother.

Francis, with his love for architecture in overdrive, was awestruck and completely thrilled by the forest of skyscrapers that panned out before him. He and Betty traveled through the Loop to a tall granite and steel office building on Wacker Drive where she received her award in some floor-to-ceiling glass office near the top of the building. As excited as he was about his mother's long overdue honor, what he remembers most is gluing his face to the plate glass window, drinking in the extraordinary view of downtown Chicago all around him. The trip was bittersweet for Betty. When she and Bob were first married, they often took their firstborn son Andrew there. Francis could easily sense this when his mother was slipping into the past. Her sadness, revealed by the faraway look in her eyes when she went to that heartbreaking place, was palpable.

A Miniature Aviator

In between school and surgeries was when Francis developed his love affair with airplanes that became an outright obsession. First, he began to meticulously draw them with astonishing accuracy, which soon progressed to building models, some of which even managed to fly or at least tried to. The most memorable time he ever spent with his father were the hours they spent, just the two of them, for the entire summer, building a model of an Eastern Airlines Lockheed L-1011 Tristar, a jumbo jet with three engines. To this day, the time they shared together remains Francis's most precious memory of his father. He still has the model airplane.

Francis's love and fascination with airplanes didn't stop there. From that point on, he wanted to learn absolutely everything he possibly could about airplanes, beyond just their physical attributes. The local library became his favorite stomping ground where he would sit and read for hours or check out any book he could on the subject.

Everyone in the family knew what to get him for birthdays and Christmas—model airplanes.

One of Francis's most exciting memories was when Betty took Ruth, James, Christopher, and Francis to visit Baer Field Airport in Fort Wayne. Baer Field, at that time, only had a small brick terminal with four ground-level gates and two jetways upstairs for jets. In those days, there was a three-sided "glass box" with a glass ceiling on the ramp level where one could get a one-hundred-eighty-degree view of the ramp as well as the sky. For more than an hour, the five of them sat there watching the big jets and small regional airplanes arrive and depart. Passengers departed by large and small numbers through the gates in the glass box. No one enjoyed the airport visit nearly as much as Francis did.

Even members of their church got in on Francis's airplane excitement. In the winter of 1988, a church member, Al Myers, took him up for a ride in his six-seat Piper. James and Pastor Smith also went along. They took off from DeKalb County Airport in Auburn and flew all over DeKalb and Steuben Counties, even doing a touch-and-go at Angola's Tri-State Airport before returning to Auburn. At that time, he had no inkling that this first flight would lead to a lifetime of traveling on many adventures by air.

A Constant Whirlwind of Smiths

These few years spent at Faith Christian Academy were a whirlwind for the Smiths. Most exciting to the entire family was the constant forward motion the Smith children were experiencing. In the fall of 1987, Becky began her first year of college at Word of Life Bible Institute at Schroon Lake in upstate New York. Francis spent much of the long scenic drive with his nose stuck to the window, drinking in every aspect of the Appalachian Mountains and the beautiful scenery that constantly unfolded before them. Which of the siblings was more excited, Becky or Francis, was difficult to say.

The Bible Institute campus was situated on the majestic Schroon Lake among the mountains of New York, a peaceful and rather isolated part of the state. The family stayed at the quaint little hotel on campus, which was where Ruth picked up her passion for napkin folding, something she remains quite the expert at today. There, the family endured numerous welcome talks from speakers who managed to put Francis to sleep. But the highlight was an exquisite wooden chapel they attended for service. There was also a fabulous recreation center with an enormous pool that everyone but Francis swam in. Their next visit there was to bring Becky back home for Christmas. This journey was even more splendid than their first as Francis watched the vision of the snowcapped mountains pass them by.

The family did not make the long trek back to upstate New York again until Becky graduated in 1988. To celebrate her wonderful achievement, they combined the visit with a family vacation on the East Coast where they camped in Pennsylvania. On the way back, they visited relatives in New Jersey where they spent a day strolling along the Boardwalk and wading in the Atlantic Ocean. This marked the first time most of them had ever seen the ocean, and it was one of their most unforgettable moments. Francis clearly remembers gazing upon the endless ocean from the seashore, feeling awestruck by his closeness to God and His majesty, a sensation that was so strong it was almost palpable. Words really cannot describe the omnipresence of God the Father, but in that moment, Francis was completely enveloped in it.

On the last leg home, the Smiths visited an unusual drive-through zoo that they all found amazing. With the windows up, of course. The closer they got to home, the more excited Francis became. Now that he was a graduate of Faith Christian Academy, he would begin his seventh-grade year at Garrett Junior-Senior High School.

Chapter 3

The Road to Perdition
1988

A Perfect Storm

Francis's memories from Faith Christian Academy were bittersweet. While his siblings all had uplifting different experiences, he had taken with him forever his strong and encouraging relationship with Keith Wittebols, but that was only one part of a larger picture, one in which he had suffered some serious setbacks and disappointments. What Francis could not understand yet, and unseen by his parents and siblings, was that through his trials at the academy, he was developing a strong backbone. He had no idea back then that God was busily preparing him all along for the terrible trials that were farther away in his unseen future.

Around this time, another trial was brewing. What Betty and Bob had managed to keep from their family was that Bob's health was failing. It was subtle at first, but more and more, Bob was not joining the family on some of their longer expeditions together. No matter how strong Betty's love for Bob was, her one disappointment was that he was a heavy smoker. He was addicted actually. His many attempts to quit had failed time and time again, and over the years, the damage caused by his smoking was irreversible by the time he finally did quit. But the children weren't really aware of this yet. It was simply accepted that their dad didn't join them because he had to work. Nothing more was ever said. Through God's grace, Betty was able to endure her torment, alone.

Garrett Junior-Senior High School

The beginning of Francis's years at Garrett Junior-Senior High School started on a positive note, and he was very excited. Garrett was much larger, plus his individual subjects each had a different teacher who resided over their own separate classrooms. Francis and Betty had visited the school prior to his first day in order to get him signed up for the core classes of social studies, math, English, and health science as well as a series of six weeklong rotation classes of cooking, woodshop, crafts, and typing. When it came to music classes though, Bob and Betty could not understand their son's reluctance to join the band, but after several long persuading talks, he eventually acquiesced.

Thankfully, Francis's parents were correct in encouraging their son back into band. Mr. Marlow was demanding, but he had the patience with the students to help them through challenging music, plus he genuinely cared about the students. For the next two years, Francis was the "jack of all trades" in the percussion section, playing everything from the bass drum to the kettledrum and onto the marimba. Several times a year, the band put on several public performances that Francis enjoyed participating in. All in all, it was a positive experience that more than made up for his previous unhappy experience.

***

For whatever reason, Betty had had the forethought to teach Francis typing. For his Christmas present in 1983, he was gifted with a toy typewriter that only typed capital letters on which he first learned to type. Eventually, when he entered typing class in junior high where he experienced his first electric typewriter, an IBM Selectric. By that time, Francis was way ahead of the game. As he became more comfortable at typing without looking at the keys for guidance, his typing speed became fast and accurate, and by the time he reached high school, he was an excellent typist.

Francis thrived in woodshop where the class made decorative miniature wooden sleds that were sold in Garrett. In cooking class, he successfully made a batch of cookies by himself. He was fascinated by all the artifacts of the kitchen that chefs mastered along with cooking techniques. In crafts, his long delicate fingers were perfect for the intricacies of latch-hook crossword-puzzle design on his homemade pillow. In eighth-grade metal shop, he made a scoop that came in handy for the dry dog food at home.

He also took an introductory computer class. In sewing, he made a beautiful blue striped apron for Susie who was engaged to marry the next summer. He joined the spelling team because spelling had always been one of his strong suits. Aside from math, where he sometimes struggled, his grades were high, and he showed a strong competitive spirit by his willingness to compete in whatever area he was good at. He even won a school geography bee, beating out the previous champ. Academically, Francis was at his zenith. With a stellar record of straight As, he made the honor roll every quarter and was the darling of all his teachers.

The Big Bad Bullies

While Francis remained popular with his teachers, he wasn't all that well-liked by his peers. Obviously, his disabilities and strange appearance set him apart, but one can only imagine how his academic success and favoritism with his teachers must have rankled some of the other students who weren't doing so well.

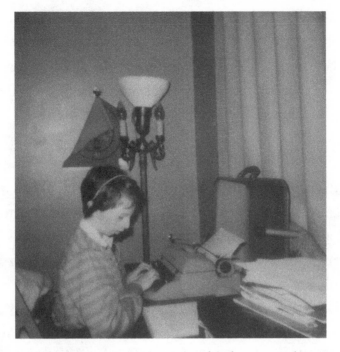

The typist. Francis typing his homework.

The trouble began in the late fall of Francis's seventh-grade year, right before Christmas vacation, 1988. It began innocuously, more or less, by some "innocent" teasing and demeaning remarks that he chose to ignore. Ignorance, he soon learned, did nothing to tone down the situation. Upon returning to school after the New Year in 1989, the bullies turned up the heat. Determined to break him, the situation soon developed into a daily unwelcomed event that was amazingly underneath the radar of the faculty and staff. At first, the abuse was only verbal, and it happened both inside as well as outside of the classrooms.

Failing to get the required response from their prey, the bullies escalated the situation. The first time Francis felt himself truly succumb to his very frightened feelings was when a ring of students circled him and ganged up on him. Before long, this torture began on a daily basis. The bullies terrorized him in the school hallways and outside on the sidelines of the playground, away from the supervising sight of the staff. The bullies wouldn't stop until they elicited an angry reaction out of him or, worse, until he started to cry. They pulled any reason out of a hat they could use to tease him, the number one reason being his facial appearance. He was most often referred to as "wax dummy." *Everything* became a target, from his expertise at difficult crossword puzzles to his being a "nerd" or the "teachers' pet." Nothing was off-limits.

But what really terrified Francis was a small group of the offenders who had become fascinated by Satanism. They were the ones who truly panicked him. They would shove him against the lockers in the hallway, frightening him beyond belief. One actually sneered in his face he was going to be sacrificed to the devil while the rest of them laughed. Francis was so terrified by this evil group he couldn't sleep at night. Once, a mother from Mothers Against Drunk Driving came to the school to speak about drinking and drunk driving. In the center of the auditorium was a casket. One of the offenders whispered in his ear, "That's *your* casket."

The bullying filled Francis with dread and terror. Most of the torment occurred in the hallways. Between classes, he became so frightened he would shake. There was safety in numbers, so he would try to attach himself to any group of students he could, only to have them try to get away from him as quickly as possible, leaving him vulnerable again. It wasn't uncommon for him to be zinged with a spitball in the back of his head or to have one of the offenders walk by and flick him in the face with his fingers, which stung. Once, he opened his locker and the books inside had been stacked, so they fell out and hit him when he opened his locker. Another time, his locker was filled to the brim with whipped cream. They stopped at nothing. He clung to the teachers whenever he could, but there were places like the instrument closet in the band room where he was immediately cornered the moment he went in to get or put his instrument away.

One day, the bullies pinned Francis to his locker. They surrounded him, verbally taunting him. Ruth happened to come by. When she saw what was happening, she quickly sprang into action. She yelled at them to leave him alone and let him go! One look at the ferocious Ruth, a double amputee powering herself along in her wheelchair with her well-muscled arms, got their attention. They quickly disbanded and ran off.

That night, Ruth told Betty what she had seen. Bob was traveling at the time. Furious, she marched into the principal's office the next day, demanding that he put an immediate stop to it. His unconcerned reply was "If your son would just quit wearing that Walkman of his, maybe the kids would give him more respect." He was referring to the large hearing aid with its headband Francis was wearing. Betty let loose on him unlike she had never let loose on anyone before in her life. Her son was referred to the school counselor.

"Francis kept all of this to himself," Betty sorrowfully remembered. "He never shared any of what was going on with us. He never ratted on any of the kids."

The school administration did absolutely nothing to alleviate the situation. Francis stayed close to his teachers who were only too happy to have him in their fold. The teachers, of course, were terribly upset by all of it. Some had actually heard rumors to the effect that he was being bullied, but none of them stepped up to help him out. Ironically, it was his easy relationships with adults that were partly responsible for his troubles, as the other kids didn't like it.

Perhaps, trying to save face, all Betty and Bob heard after that incident was "Francis just doesn't fit in. He's too smart for any of them. He doesn't belong here." The bullying finally did come to a stop, but the psychological and the emotional scars he formed have never really completely healed to this day.

Inferno

By the end of two years, the damage was complete. Before middle school, Francis had been a relatively happy, active little boy. The hurt began early in fifth grade by the unacceptance of his peers and the ongoing anger from his band teacher, an adult who should have known better. He singlehandedly nearly destroyed his love of music. But that paled by comparison in junior and senior high school when some of his peers sadly displayed exactly what they were capable of and how far they would go to provoke a terrified reaction from him.

In order to survive, Francis quickly learned to bury his feelings deep inside of himself and to develop a tough, hard, cold exterior. The joy in living his life was gone. He became a zombie who went through the motions of life, refusing along the way to participate in anything. For solace, he buried himself deeply into his beloved collection of toy airplanes where he spent hours upon hours playing with them, alone. At one time, riding his bike around the block with his sister Ruth in hot pursuit had been his favorite pastime. Now the bike sat in the garage, unused, and no amount of coaxing could get him to take it out and ride it.

Never before in Francis's short young life had he felt so alone. Even his love for his LORD was to no avail. God couldn't help him because Francis wouldn't let Him. His young Christian faith was shattered, but somehow, it was still there. He was in a state of deep isolation and loneliness.

The Smiths did everything they could possibly do to reach out to him, but none of them was capable of realizing the depth of their son's despair. He was completely demoralized and emotionally dead.

A Frightening Illness

By the summer of 1990, Francis began to suffer from the strange malady of not being able to keep his food down, which led to his becoming dangerously malnourished and subsequently emaciated. It was assumed that his emotional trauma had manifested itself into a serious illness.

Horrified and frightened, Betty took him to the dietician at Riley Hospital. She was advised to *immediately* put Francis on a diet of high calories, milk, half-and-half cream, fatty foods, and anything else that would put weight onto him. Much to everyone's horror, he couldn't keep any of it down, and the illness only got worse, and before long, his frame was dangerously skeletal. It wasn't until much later that he was actually diagnosed as lactose intolerant and allergic to milk. The very foods that were used in hopes of helping him gain some weight and get better were actually making him even sicker. At last, by eliminating dairy from his diet, his alarming plummeting weight loss began to subside. Through even this ordeal, Francis's ongoing turmoil was still in evidence.

The Karate Kid

Grasping at straws, the Riley Hospital referred the Smiths to the Turnstone Center for Disabled Children and Adults in Fort Wayne, where there was a counselor who worked with other children with bullying and self-esteem issues. Betty and Francis attended the meetings for a few weeks, but he was unable to express what he was going through. Unwilling to give up in getting help for her son, Betty signed him up for karate lessons.

In early 1990, Bob found a karate school that was run by a police officer, Randy Duhamell, who specialized in the Korean martial art of tae kwon do. Francis was introduced to his *sensei* (teacher), Officer Duhamell, and was issued his own small-sized *ghee* (uniform) complete with white belt, padded gloves, and boots. But, over a period of six months, he only progressed to his yellow belt. His painfully slow progress was partly due to his time constraints, but mostly, it was because of his poor gross-motor muscular coordination. Despite everyone's best intentions, karate proved much too difficult for him to master and only managed to add another level of frustration for all concerned.

The Struggle for Survival

The bottom line was Francis's life was irrevocably changed. Gone was his innocence, a life that was filled by people who loved, cared, and advocated for him. Although those loving people still existed in his life, his heart and psyche were now badly scarred by the reality of the very real hatred and wickedness that existed deep inside the human heart and soul and the knowledge that there was just so much others could do to help him. The world was a very cruel place, and sooner or later, he would have to learn to survive on his own.

Decades later in 2012, after he achieved his PhD in oral and craniofacial sciences, Francis put his thoughts into an open letter on the editorial page of the Fort Wayne *News Sentinel,* in hopes of making the public aware of the personal pain and dangers of bullying and also to express his personal experience. Here is a copy of this letter:

An Open Letter Concerning the Terror and Aftermath of Bullying
Dr. Francis Joel Smith, PhD with Michele DuBroy

During Mitt Romney's presidential campaign, the issue of his involvement in a bullying incident was brought up by some commentators and, later on, the media. When he was fifteen years old, he led other boys to hunt down and tease John Lauber, a quiet, offbeat type, who had bleached his hair blond during spring break. When they found him, the others held him pinned to the ground, no doubt terrorized while Romney cut off his hair with a pair of scissors, something he later on admitted to.

However, some of Romney's supporters chose to downplay the incident. While some people will say "kids will be kids" or that the victim can get over it quickly and "man up," none of that is true. Bullying, in fact, can have long-lasting effects on victims, scarring them for life or even leading to suicide.

Personally, I can attest to that from my own life experience with school bullying and its frightful aftermath. Because I was born with craniofacial deformities, I have always looked a lot different from others. People unfortunately tend to judge others based on their external appearance.

All through my childhood, I attended a variety of schools, both public and parochial. Because I was judged by my outward appearance, I was often kept out of class by teachers who felt that they could not handle my unique challenges. Since I had no outer ears, they falsely assumed that I could not hear. At that time, I very well could hear. The hearing device I wore was an old-fashioned, cumbersome Walkman-style device with a large battery that was strapped to my chest. I also suffered from a cleft palate and its associated speech problems. One church school actually refused admission to me at first based on that basis although one teacher became my advocate and stood up and fought for me until I was admitted.

But all of that paled by comparison as soon as I entered my junior high school years in a local public school district. There, for two years, I was subjected to endless, merciless taunting, teasing, physical abuse, and even threats of harm or death. The taunting and threats were bad enough, but before long, the situation escalated to spitwads, pushing, and even cornering me in the hallway, classrooms, or band room. One time, my younger sister, who also suffers disabilities, saw some kids backing me up against a wall of lockers in the hall. Thankfully, she bravely intervened and then told my parents who had no idea any of this was going on. As soon as my mother found out, she confronted the school principal, demanding that he put a stop to it. His reply? "If he would take off that ridiculous-looking Walkman, maybe the kids would respect him." Mom was livid, I can imagine. That so-called "Walkman" was my bone conduction hearing aid that was held to my head with a headband.

Every day at school became more and more torturous. Somehow, I managed to survive by learning to bury my feelings. On the outside, I was cold and hard, giving the appearance that I was just going through the motions of life. On the inside, I could no longer feel anything or relate to anyone; I was one of the living dead. It was a living hell. My parents had no idea what was really going on, as

I hid everything inside. It even affected me physically and spiritually. I felt totally alone. Only God carried me through this terrible phase of my life. It was not until I transferred to Canterbury School in Fort Wayne for high school (where I encountered acceptance for the first time) that I was able to embark on the long road to recovery.

Bullying oftentimes scars for life. Please—I implore you. Never turn away from a child, teen, or a special needs person who is being bullied. Intervention can save that person from a lifetime of torment and pain.

Sincerely,
Dr. Francis Joel Smith

A Gradual Healing of Sorts

Around this time, other people who suffered from Treacher Collins syndrome managed to surface in his life. Once, while visiting the craniofacial outpatient clinic at Riley Hospital, Francis became acquainted with a young professional with the same severity of the syndrome that he had. His name was John Smyser, and the two of them hit it off from the first time they met. While they did not exactly socialize, they kept in touch through letters, and they both considered their friendship a solid one. Occasionally, they ran into each other at Riley Hospital, and later on, they both attended Camp About Face. One of the highlights of that week for Francis was the big beach party at the lake where the campers got to socialize with Riley Hospital doctors, professionals, and some of the sponsors of the program (e.g., the Jaycees). It was a grand picnic complete with games, hamburgers, hot dogs, and barbecued chicken.

All too soon, the week at Camp About Face came to an end. Bob, Betty, and Ruth came down to pick Francis up. All the way home, Ruth regaled Francis endlessly with her latest experience and asked him nonstop questions about the camp. It seemed they were home in no time. This time, Francis practically kissed the ground in front of their house. No more mosquitoes!

Francis loved these camps, and later on, get-togethers such as these would become an ongoing fixture in his life. They not only instilled in him the need to be with others who were challenged, as he was, he also received great joy in being able to encourage others and to share in their growth and successes. Besides, he made many lifelong friends in the craniofacial community.

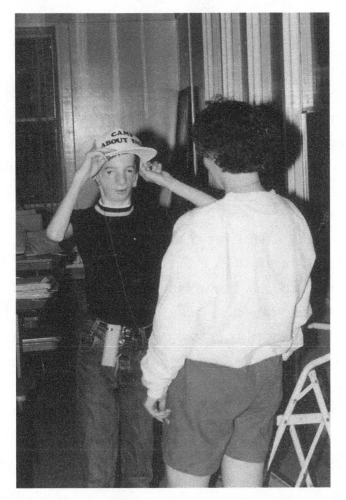

Francis overcame many challenges
while at Camp About Face.

Rising from the Ashes

Once back home, Francis's life continued to move forward. Under the tutelage of his piano teacher Marquita Kelsey, he was prepared to participate in the annual piano recitals. Betty actually taped one of the recitals, and during one of their many forays back to Riley Hospital where he underwent ongoing dental and craniofacial checkups, they always planned to visit Mrs. Collins in the inner city. Mrs. Collins was still very much a part of their lives, and after listening to the tape of Francis's piano playing, she was reduced to tears. Thankfully, Betty and Francis spared her from ever knowing that he had been bullied. It would have devastated her.

An Ever-changing Family

Over time, the Smith family began to dwindle in size, and nowhere was that reflected more than during the family camping trips. Since the Smiths always traveled by motor, camping was a way of life. Whereas the older boys would help Bob set up the trailer, now it became Francis's job. He would help hook the trailer to the van, set it up, jack it up, and carry out the other heavy chores. Right after Camp About Face, Bob, Betty, Francis, and Ruth took a two-week drive out to Illinois, Iowa, and Nebraska. Their first stop was for a few days in Galesburg, Illinois, to see Aunt Stewie, their first visit with her since their most memorable Christmas. She had not yet met Ruth, and they took a terrific liking to each other.

Along the way, they camped at Story Lake, then onto Bishop Hill where they visited a restored Swedish colony. On the way back home, they stopped to visit Betty's brother, Bobbie Johnson, in Modale, Iowa. Betty and her brother Bobbie could not have been more unalike. Where

Betty abided in her lifelong faith that was deeply instilled in her during the Great Depression, Bobbie swore he would never be subjected to those terrible conditions again. He drove himself to succeed and was now an extremely wealthy businessman. But even though he had riches, he was running on empty. The joy and peace that sustained his sister through her years of trials completely evaded him. Although their sibling bonds were secure, Betty and her brother had very little in common.

Before heading west and back home, the Smiths swung by their great-aunt Dorothy from Betty's side of the family. Traveling back through Illinois, they stopped in New Salem, a village where Abraham Lincoln spent a portion of his young adulthood, as well has his home in Springfield, where he is now buried. None of them knew it, but this would be the last family vacation they would take together. Bob's health was failing.

I will never leave nor forsake you.
—Hebrews 13:5

As for you, you meant evil against me,
but God meant it for good,
to bring it about that many people
should be kept alive,
as they are today.
—Genesis 50:20

What Man Intends for Evil…

There were other big changes in the family during Francis's junior high school years. James sadly gave in to the devastation of his drug addiction that was inflicted upon him at birth. Unable to form stable and lasting relationships, he was prone to outbursts that were brought on by no fault of his own. But action reaps consequences, and as he got older, he got in with the wrong crowd. He finally gave in to his body's natural craving for drugs and, in short order, found himself dealing drugs that led him into trouble with the law. Not surprising to anyone, he ended up in jail, only this was just the first of several incarcerations that lurked in his future. Bob and Betty were naturally devastated. That didn't make them love him any less. If anything, they were thankful that for as long as he was incarcerated, at least he was away from others who led him to harm—for a while, that is. This was the beginning of a vicious cycle where he would be behind bars, be released, only to get mixed up with the wrong people again and end up back in jail. The victorious story of their son Peter, who had also landed in hot water several years prior, gave them hope and faith that someday, through the intervention of their LORD, James would be able to overcome his terrible bondage of addiction. Someday, that would happen. But for now, this was a terribly difficult and painful time for all of them. Visits to the jail to see James were something they would all partake in, which he wholeheartedly appreciated. This was a case of his addiction overtaking the desires of his heart. He wasn't strong yet.

God Intends for Good

But James knew the LORD, and he began to lean steadily on Him. His family was loving and loyal. Both Bob and Betty had a great peace in the midst of their sorrow for James that this was where the LORD wanted him, and through his incarcerations, the LORD was not only protecting him from the very outside sources he was still so weak against; He was also doing His best work in their son's life. James was exactly where the LORD wanted him.

James

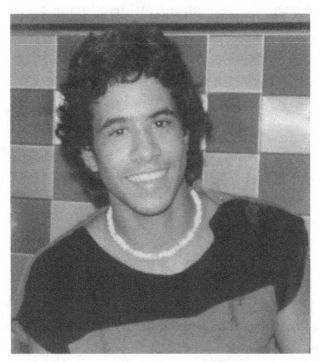

James's renewed faith in the LORD
would eventually reap victory.

Love Is in the Air

On a happy note, Susie had fallen in love! While she was attending Auburn Missionary Church, she had met and fallen in love with the love of her life, and he proposed to her. The Smiths held the rehearsal dinner at their home. Even though their wedding day was a gray and rainy day, the joy of their love shone through. On Susie's wedding day, she walked proudly down the aisle on Bob's arm, completely unaided in any other way. Bob and her brothers were resplendent in their tuxedoes. The bride, her mother, and her sisters were beautiful in their long gowns. Among the wedding gifts was an apron, handmade and sewn by Francis. It was a joyous occasion.

The following spring, on Mother's Day, Betty was honored in a unique way. She was invited to speak at a church in Van Wert, Ohio. While Francis played "Were You There" on the piano, Christopher sang along in his rich baritone voice. Afterward, the pastor invited them to his beautiful Victorian home for dinner.

The Last Adoption

After many years of being permanent foster children, the adoptions of Francis and Ruth were, at last, finalized.

During a formal court hearing at the DeKalb County Court House in Auburn, the Honorable Judge Paul Cherry had Bob and Betty sign the adoption papers as Francis and Ruth sat on the witness bench. Francis's and Ruth's caseworkers were there as witnesses, and so was James who was released from jail just for this day so he could be a witness too. As soon as the adoption papers were signed, His Honor came from behind his desk and posed for a family photo. The adoption process for Francis, and later on Ruth, had dragged on for so many years. Their official status had been "permanent foster placement" as opposed to true adoption. Bob and Betty had wanted, all along, to adopt both of them, but one of the many issues that stood in the way were the medical bills. As long as they were fostered, they had assistance. But after years of red tape, Bob was able to prove his reliability along with his ability to pay for their medical bills through his insurance and income. Their official adoption was the happiest day of Francis's and Ruth's lives.

The happiest day.

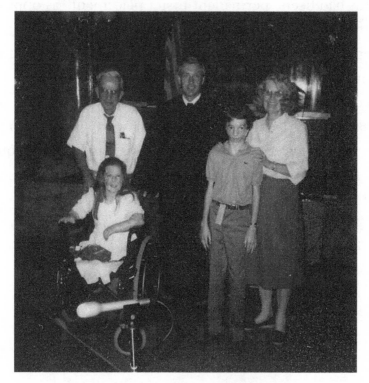

The Smiths with the judge after
Francis's and Ruth's adoption.

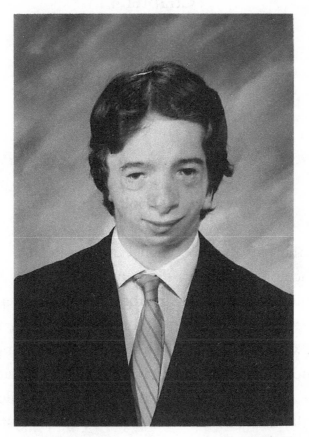

Francis's freshman portrait, Canterbury High School.
He still had several facial reconstructive
surgeries in his future.

Chapter 4

Let the Healing Begin
1989

A New High School: Acceptance

In the fall of 1989 when Francis was in the eighth grade, he noticed an advertisement in *The Evening Star* that would ultimately turn his life around. A small independent college-preparatory school, Canterbury School, in Fort Wayne, was running a high school scholarship competition for eighth graders. He brought the article to the attention of Bob and Betty. Knowing that their son was desperate for an alternative to the Garrett public school system and believing in his capabilities, they encouraged him to give it his all. The next day, Betty contacted Canterbury School and set up a reservation for the scholarship competition test.

On the first Saturday of that November, Betty, Bob, and Francis went to the Canterbury High School campus. Nestled deeply in a bucolic, woodsy setting and completely isolated from the bustling subdivisions and strip malls of southwest Fort Wayne, it felt set apart and deeply inviting to all of them. The headmaster's home was also on site, just a brief walk to the school.

Francis was introduced to one of the staff that was there to administer the extensive battery of tests for the scholarship competition. The Smiths were rather taken aback at the large number of students that showed up. Most of them were from Canterbury Middle School, but there were others, like Francis, who arrived from other schools.

For the next several hours, the students battled a rigorous battery of examinations in math and English. Bob and Betty used that time to talk with the high school administration and other staff about their son concerning his expectations, past experiences, and goals. After Francis completed the tests, all the prospective students were taken on a tour of the campus by some of the teachers. The auditorium was complete with a stage. The cafeteria was large, and the locker accommodations were spacious. The library itself was of special interest to Francis, as were the biology, physics, and chemistry labs along with the computer classroom. Outside were the tennis courts and soccer fields. They attended a presentation in the auditorium about the school and were given a thick folder of information. Needless to say, Francis, Bob, and Betty were beside themselves with excitement.

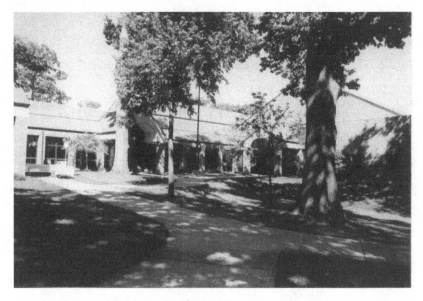

Image: Courtesy of Ruth Smith
Canterbury High School, where the healing began.

Hopes Dashed

A few weeks later, the high school administration called with the results of Francis's examination. Francis had failed to win a scholarship.

After the disappointment sank in, Bob and Betty were surprised to learn that Francis was being offered a partial tuition scholarship for the duration of high school. Evidently, everyone was so impressed by his story and life experiences along with his own personal fortitude they were inspired to offer him a partial scholarship!

Right before Christmas break, the high school administration reached out and invited Francis to visit the campus for a day and sit in on all the classes he would be attending the next year as a freshman. They met with the headmaster, Mr. Hancock, for the first time. An English native, he was an Oxford man, complete with the accent, demeanor, and appearance to go with it. Francis was so excited to spend the entire day as a "regular" student. He wasn't the least bit shy about walking into the classrooms and settling in. The stares didn't bother him. Actually, they were minimal, and several students took it upon themselves to welcome him into their classes. There was curiosity, but there was none of the hostility or animosity he had experienced so often in the past. The atmosphere was inviting.

Francis was totally captivated by each teacher and their individual classrooms. Biology was taught by a big bear of a man, Mr. King, who had a very warm temperament. Francis remembers Mr. King's lesson to this day; he lectured on the internal pressure of cells being affected by the concentration of solids in the liquid environment. Francis was fascinated.

Moving on to the English department, his new teacher just happened to be the headmaster's wife. Mrs. Hancock was tall, thin, silver haired, and elegant. What made her of utmost interest was her passion for teaching various forms of literary work—poetry, short stories, and novels—with an emphasis on the study of literature and creative writing. In algebra, he encountered Mr. Furiak, whose boundless enthusiasm for the subject was contagious. For world history, Dr. Werhli engaged in an incredible discussion of ancient Mesopotamian history. Then there was the French teacher, Mrs. Gerber. Petite and dark haired, her enthusiasm for the language and culture completely captivated him. Because of her, he chose to study French over the other two languages, Spanish and Latin.

The LORD, without fail, had intervened once again; and Francis, Betty, and Bob were ecstatic!

An Exciting Summer

The powers that be at Canterbury did not waste any time preparing Francis for the upcoming school year. He was given a lengthy required reading list for English that included Tolkien's *The Hobbit* from the *Lord of the Rings* series, Malamud's *The Natural*, Douglas Adams's *The Hitchhiker's Guide to the Galaxy*, and many others. Every summer from that point on during his high school years would be filled with required reading for the coming year. Francis didn't mind. He loved to read, and he couldn't think of a better way to occupy his time.

But nothing prepared him for the gift that was yet to come. That summer, Francis got the first opportunity to meet his freshman classmates. The freshman introduction party was held at the upscale Fort Wayne home of the family of one of the students. It was a great evening. Right away, Francis noticed something different about these students. They had fun together. They were serious about their schooling, and none of them hesitated to reach out to him and accept him just as he was. There was a certain maturity and openness about them he had never experienced among his peers before. Instead of just looking at the physical appearance of someone, they were able to see one another for the unique person each one of them truly was. Not knowing what to expect, he was pleasantly surprised, and for the first time in his life, he was able to reach out and enjoy his fellow students.

Francis's peers reached out to him in many ways. One memorable example was that just before Francis turned sixteen, one of the girls in his class stayed up all night in her kitchen at home baking a beautiful birthday cake for him, which was shared by everyone at school the next day for his birthday.

A Dynamic Workload

From the first day of school, Francis quickly discovered that Canterbury High was unlike any other learning institution he had attended, and he loved it. Each morning, the entire school assembled together for nonsectarian chapel in the auditorium for school announcements along with either a performance of some kind or a message that was given by a teacher or a guest speaker. Once, in his freshman year, Francis gave a solo piano performance of *The Russian Concerto* by Sergei Rachmaninoff. On another occasion, members of the Fort Wayne Philharmonic Orchestra gave a performance and then explained what it was like to play in a professional orchestra. At Christmas, Mr. King, the biology teacher, organized his entire class into a choir. They performed *Dona Nobis Pacem*. At Thanksgiving and Christmas, the entire school gathered at the lower and middle school campus on Covington Road for an all-school chapel and meal. This was always a welcomed great way to start off the school day; the purpose of this morning time together was to instill proper ethics and moral values in a Judeo-Christian vein as well as to expose the students to a rich diversity of cultures and arts.

The new way of learning didn't stop there. The students were taught to take pride in their school. At the end of the school day, the students gathered into their respective work crews to clean up. One of Francis's group duties was to vacuum, clean chalkboards and erasers, and stow audiovisual equipment away.

Dress code was also of utmost importance, and still to this day, Francis takes great care in the way he dresses. On Wednesdays, the boys wore shirts and ties, and girls were required to wear dresses or skirts. The Wednesday dress code was not a suggestion—it was mandatory. One Wednesday morning, Francis forgot. He came to school in a shirt with no tie, only to be confronted by all the other students who had complied. Improvising on the spot so he wouldn't get a demerit, he grabbed an orange cleaning rag and tucked into the collar of his shirt. It was an "ugly tie," complete with cleaning stains, but perhaps everyone simply thought he ate a sloppy breakfast. Regardless, he avoided being sent home with a demerit.

Not the least bit surprising, the biggest shock to his system of all was Francis was loaded to the gills with both class and homework. Normally, he was in bed fast asleep each night by nine. It didn't take long for him to figure out that that wasn't nearly enough time to get his home-work done. Within weeks, he was pulling all-nighters, and Mountain Dew with its high caffeine became his loyal study companion. For some reason, he reveled in the challenge, and his grades reflected his hard work. Actually, he loved it. No one ever heard him complain.

It was during Francis's freshman year that Jill Krementz, a children's author from New York City, approached the Smiths about including his personal story in a book she was writing about children with various physical disabilities. Riley Hospital and their craniofacial community had brought Francis's plight to her attention. Ms. Krementz asked him if he would write a chapter about his own story. Mrs. Hancock, his English teacher, also rose to this monumental occasion by using this assignment as an opportunity to help Francis express many suppressed and buried feelings. This proved to be an extremely difficult challenge for him as only one year had passed since junior high, and the pain and terror of his being bullied was still very raw. By spring, with Mrs. Hancock's help, he was able to submit the written chapter to Ms. Krementz.

For an entire day, the two of them sat in the speech therapy office where he and Trish Severns were inter-viewed. Eventually, she went on to interview Bob and Betty, his doctors, and even the school headmaster. During her time at the camp, she managed to take several wonder-ful black-and-white photos of Francis at camp, including one of him paddling a canoe. Other campers and counsel-ors got to know her, and one of the favorite topics among them was about the previous books she had written.

One year later, *How It Feels to Live with a Physical Disability* was published. One of Francis's prized possessions is the original copy she sent him in the mail. He was now a published author. Some of the daily papers in Fort Wayne, Auburn, and Indianapolis got wind of the story; and all of a sudden, they were all publishing their own accounts of Francis's life story. He found himself to be a bit of a celebrity, complete with autographing copies of the book in his town's library and, later, the university library. What a turnaround the LORD had orchestrated, barely two years from the crippling experience of being bullied. One can only wonder what the reaction was of those who had wittingly or unwittingly taken part in causing him so much harm.

A Most Serious Surgery

Within two years at Canterbury High and much to the delight and relief of Francis's family, his life had done a complete turnaround. The pain from the bullying was still with him as it was a life-altering experience. But it had lost its ugly grip on him, and he was finally experiencing what they had all hoped for: an acceptance and admiration among his peers for who he was and his outstanding accomplishments and contributions in the school community.

With this new security along with his growing maturity firmly in place, Francis had to face the most serious and difficult surgery of his life. In order to normalize his facial structure, an oral-maxillofacial surgery was necessary. His lower jaw was to be rebuilt using rib grafts that would require that his jaw be wired shut for two months. A temporary trach would enable him to breathe during that time.

The process began in November 1991 at Riley Hospital where Francis had his final checkup and preparations for the surgery, including giving a pint of his own blood should an autotransfusion be necessary. The surgery was scheduled for December 4, so in order to prepare for his absence, he collected his textbooks and makeup work that would enable him to stay current with his rigorous academic classes.

The night before the surgery, Betty and Francis packed up the Chevy station wagon for the trip down to Indianapolis. In the dark of that December night, they started driving down Interstate 69. Feeling very tired, Betty and Francis decided to pull into a rest stop for a quick nap. What an unfortunate decision. They must have been very tired, for they both slept straight through for several hours. Snow was not expected that night, but when they awoke, they were both half frozen, and the car was practically buried. After finally digging themselves out, they began the long slow drive down the snow-drifted Interstate 69 in whiteout blizzard conditions. By some miracle, they finally made it to Indianapolis in time for check-in at Riley at four thirty in the morning.

After being prepped for the surgery and the final blood test was drawn, Dr. Nelson and Dr. Hayhurst, along with the anesthesiologist, came into his cubicle to discuss what the surgery would entail. After a hug goodbye to Betty, Francis was walked through the double doors.

Once Francis was put to sleep with the mask and an IV and after a tracheostomy was done, the fourteen hours of surgery began. The surgeons cut his lower jaw on both sides. Two pieces of rib with cartilage end caps were harvested and used to make new ball joints on each side. In order to align his jaw in a new orientation whereby the teeth would be closer together, screws were used to fasten it all together. The upper and lower jaws were wired together for the next two months.

Francis awoke in recovery with a tracheostomy and his jaws wired tightly together. He had a catheter in his bladder and a stomach tube to remove blood from his stomach and to keep it clear. His hair was full of blood, as he had lost quite a bit during the surgery; his mother would be washing it out of his hair for days after he got home. Once he was awake, he was wheeled into intensive care unit (ICU) because of the tracheostomy and his need for oxygen.

The ICU was where he almost lost his life.

In the middle of the night, he awoke, unable to take in air. His trach had plugged up with phlegm. At first, he was completely paralyzed by fear, but his will to survive kicked in. He grabbed the call button and frantically pushed it. The seconds it took for the nurse to respond seemed like an eternity—for sure he was going to die. He was so frenzied the nurse had to pin him down with one hand while she struggled to get the blocked cannula removed so she could suction him. Just on the verge of blacking out, he began to gulp in the air. He had never been so terrified in his life, certain he was going to die of asphyxiation. The experience so rattled him he was afraid to fall asleep again. Fortunately, everything ran smoothly after that, and he was no longer required to remain in the ICU.

Due to a lack of rooms, Francis was moved to the isolation room in the teen unit. Actually, that was a relief because, when he had visitors, no one had to worry about disturbing others, and his visits were much more relaxed. After a few more days, his stomach tube and catheter were removed, and he was able to begin a thin liquid diet of juice and broth, delivered by a large syringe with a short rubber hose on the nozzle.

Eventually, Francis regained his strength enough to walk around. He loved going to the Riley Family Library in the older part of the hospital, run by another lovely woman who had befriended him years before, Lynn Dunnagan. She was very much a mother to him, and he loved spending time with her. He also liked to visit the teen unit recreation room where he used the time to catch up on makeup assignments from Canterbury.

Dr. Nelson liked to drop by along with other doctors and nurses to check up on him. One day, Francis was wheeled through the underground tunnels from Riley Hospital over to the oral surgery clinic in the basement of Long Hospital, where Dr. Nelson and his colleagues closely examined their handiwork.

Eight days later, Francis was released to go home. Somehow, a carload of medical equipment that included feeding syringes, tracheostomy tubes and supplies, plus a hefty suction machine were packed inside the station wagon. Although Christmas vacation was only days away, and against his doctor's wishes, he was determined to return to school and get back into the groove as quickly as possible. He also wanted to take the semester finals, much to everyone's surprise.

An Unexpected Honor

Completely unsuspecting of the high regard in which he was held, Francis walked into the school auditorium on the morning he returned only to be greeted by a standing ovation! Hanging from the wall outside the auditorium was a huge banner, WELCOME BACK, FRANCIS! He was completely overwhelmed and nearly moved to tears.

In the classrooms, teachers and students reached out to him and did everything they could in order to make sure he was comfortable. In his English class, a student named Elizabeth Armbuster became his personal guardian angel. She let him know right away that she was there for him should he need anything. A few days later, he did. Still weak from his ordeal, he struggled mightily under the weight of the many books he carried in his backpack. One morning, he literally fell over in the hall, the books spilling onto the floor. Before he could even stand, she was by his side. She knelt beside him and helped him pick up his books, then carried the backpack herself to his next class. She rose to the challenge on several different times between then and Christmas, an act of kindness he remembers to this day. It was the first time he was ever cared so deeply for by a peer. Until then, he had only faced the cruelty of rejection, which sadly he had stoically come to expect.

Thankfully, Francis passed his exams with flying colors in spite of not feeling completely well. At last, he was showing his true academic grit and was being rewarded mightily for it.

During a trip back to Riley Hospital for Children, the trach that irritated him so much was removed. Back home for the duration of Christmas vacation, he enjoyed Betty's magical, wonderful blenderized recipes that were hyped up a little for the holidays. The scrumptious Christmas dinner of roast beef and ham, mashed potatoes, green beans, relishes, salads, and dinner rolls that was displayed on their dining room table somehow ended up in a blender, so Francis was served his Christmas dinner through a syringe. He didn't miss a thing.

Let the Music Begin

What was affected by Francis's latest surgery was his music, which had to be put on hold for a while. Francis simply didn't have the physical stamina yet nor the energy he needed in order to play his instruments. Even though missing his lessons was disappointing, his piano teacher, Mrs. Kelsey, encouraged him to enter his first solo piano competition, put on by the Indiana State School Music Association (ISSMA) that runs the state school music ensemble and solo contests. This required him to memorize and play an approved solo. Francis placed first in his division of the district piano solo contest held at Wayne High School.

After the removal of his jaw wires the following February, Francis was able to eat solid foods again. This milestone was celebrated by a family dinner at the buffet restaurant, Laughner's Cafeteria where Francis enjoyed one of his standby favorites, spaghetti.

After a reprieve of a few months, Francis returned to Riley Hospital for the second phase of his jaw alignment surgery. This time, it was his upper jaw that would be cut apart along the side and just beneath the nose. Remembering the serious loss of blood from his lower jaw surgery, Dr. Nelson and Dr. Hayhurst recommended that he give a unit of blood to be drawn at the Fort Wayne local Red Cross so his own blood would be on hand if need be.

During this surgery, his upper jaw was cut and brought forward before fastening it in place with rib grafts and screws. Thankfully, this time there was no need for a trach. Instead of his jaws being rigidly wired together, rubber bands were placed to allow for some movement of his lower jaw. Although he was back to having some blender-ized meals, this time he could eat some soft food such as applesauce and mashed potatoes with a spoon, which was a quite welcomed improvement.

As usual, Francis took the necessary surgeries in stride, and he persevered with his ever-increasing high school workload without any complaint. What mattered was how well he was accepted not only by the faculty but now his peers as well. He wasn't an oddity anymore. He was a student who loved to learn and was diligent in achieving his best results. His ongoing struggles with math and chemistry still challenged him, but his grades remained better than passable. Francis was a respected member of his high school community.

Preparing for College

Upon his return to Canterbury High, Francis quickly discovered that the workload for his junior year, with its preparation for college, was significantly more challenging than his sophomore year had been.

Actually, Francis was delighted by his newest work challenges. There was a certain excitement that permeated this college prep year that left everyone in high spirits and with a newly charged look at the reality that their choices would soon bring them.

In physics, Mr. Furiak (again) led the class through complex experiments on momentum with the class writing detailed lab reports, complete with data and graphs.

During May term, minicourses in anatomy, Japanese, Hebrew, science fiction, and others were offered. Francis opted to study anatomy. Using a fetal pig for dissection, he kept its brain in a jar of formaldehyde as a souvenir at home, much to Betty's horror. The reality was though he was not only fascinated by this subject and excelling, he was beginning to see a career in medicine for himself. It was certainly a real possibility.

Francis also loved British literature. His instructor, Mr. Callicutt, was a tall man with black hair, who taught with a fascinating, engaging, dramatic flair the students loved. The class was instructed to write research papers on their desired British work. Francis chose Charles Dickens's *Oliver Twist*. Deeply encouraged as a budding writer, he wrote an essay on his unique life experience for an essay competition that won him a college scholarship.

Even Francis's music progressed to a new high. He joined the jazz ensemble as their pianist, and for the first time, he played the electronic keyboard during a concert in the spring of 1993. The ensemble, conducted by Mrs. Gnagey, played with a spirit of enthusiasm he had never experienced before, and because of that, he stayed with the ensemble through the end of his senior year.

This was also the year the class began to explore college campuses. The class traveled in a chartered bus down to the southeast United States to visit colleges in North and South Carolina and Georgia. They visited Wake Forest University, Warren Wilson College, Georgia Tech, and others during the course of one week.

However, in spite of the fun and challenges of his junior year, Francis still had numerous hospital visits and surgeries to face. Only now, and for the first time, he knew for certain his peers supported him. Everyone seemed to know when he was about to face another surgical "adventure," and true to Canterbury's spirit, they all stood behind him.

In March 1993, when the bus that carried the students on their junior college expedition arrived back at Canterbury, Betty was right there waiting for them. Many of the students surrounded Francis, shaking his hand, giving hugs and words of encouragement. Betty practically had to pry her son loose from his peers. Instead of heading back home, she and Francis drove straight to Indianapolis that night for his surgery the next morning.

This time, Francis was facing two different surgeries. There was a new doctor in the fold, Dr. Eppley, who was an enthusiastic young brand-new plastic surgeon. In order to fill out his sunken skull-like face, a set of custom-made bio-absorbable porous white contoured implants were inserted below each eye socket and in the chin. These implants had been custom-made especially for him by Biomet in Warsaw, Indiana, from CAT scans that had been taken of his face a month earlier. Just for assurance, a duplicate set was made that was eventually given to Francis who, it was rumored, had quite a collection of artifacts from his numerous medical procedures! The surgery was to be performed in two phases. During the second stage of the procedure, Dr. Helveston, a Riley ophthalmologist, needed to readjust the muscles of his right eye so it would not stick out so far and get irritated by his eyelashes. When he awoke from surgery, he had double vision that lasted for a few days, but he was released after an overnight stay.

The contour implant below his right eye began to cause problems almost immediately; an infection set in, and within two weeks, Betty had to take Francis back to Riley to have it checked out. Dr. Eppley immediately scheduled surgery for the next day. He surgically drained the infected site where cellulitis, caused by staphylococcus bacteria, had colonized in the implant area. This time, Francis had to stay hospitalized for one week while he underwent a course of heavy IV antibiotics.

A Milestone Birthday, Hospital Style!

Francis's unexpected hospitalization coincided with his eighteenth birthday although no one felt the least bit sorry for him. The eye-fetching nurses in the teen unit not only captivated him, they brought him a sinfully delicious chocolate cake while singing *Happy Birthday!* Actually, he was thrilled to have so much attention in such an upbeat fashion, and this birthday in particular remains one of his happiest birthday memories. Still, the IV antibiotics were taking a dreadful toll on him. The antibiotics were so strong they were destroying his veins, necessitating that the needle be removed and inserted into other veins several times, which was quite torturous. Once, a visit to the emergency room was required after the nurses unsuccessfully tried to reinsert his IV. Eventually, this latest trauma came to a close, and he was sent home with oral antibiotics with instructions to wash his mouth out with salt water daily.

Turning eighteen is a major milestone in life, one that marks the passage from being a kid into adulthood. For Francis, it was bittersweet. This also meant that this would be his last summer for Camp About Face.

As his farewell gift from his fellow campers and counselors, he received the handmade Olympic-themed flag the group had made from the previous year, which had been signed by everyone.

***

When one door closes, another door opens. From that point on, any group expedition Francis chose to participate in would be one that carried a great purpose.

That same summer, he was invited to travel on a mission trip to Mexico with his church youth group. This would entail flying on a commercial aircraft, his first, and he was beyond excited. The group started out in Indianapolis and ended up in Harlingen, Texas, where they boarded buses to cross the Mexican border. For an entire week, the group served in one of the *colonias* (shantytowns) in Matamoros. There they went to work building two simple wooden one-room houses, ran a vacation Bible school for the children, along with a makeshift medical and dental clinic in the single public building, a squat green cinderblock building. The one-hundred-degree sun beat down unmercifully on the group, hitting Francis especially hard. His white Irish skin was burnt to a crisp, and boy, oh, boy, did he get sun sick.

A church member who was a doctor with the group tended to Francis the best he could with what little he had, and somehow, he got him up and running in spite of his terrible reaction to the heat. The doctor also had some training in dental extraction, and he gave Francis the job of keeping his dental instruments and metal syringes sterile and loaded for each patient. Much to his surprise, the doctor asked him to assist him in pulling a tooth. He jumped at the chance. The poor, hapless patient, an elderly Mexican lady, sat in the white plastic chair, got her shot in the gum, and sat still while Francis stuck the forceps in her mouth. Under the doctor's guidance, he managed to find the bad tooth. He latched onto it with the forceps and wiggled it back and forth, and soon, he had the tooth out of her mouth. Someone in the group had a camera, and before anyone could say, "Cheese," she managed to take photos of him pulling the tooth and holding it in the forceps in his hand. That became the signature moment of the trip.

***

There was more excitement waiting at home. Becky, one of the twins, was getting married. A few years prior, she had fallen in love with one of her former high school classmates at Faith Christian Academy. Her beloved proposed the summer before, and now the wedding was slated to take place at the Auburn Missionary Church where they both attended. The Smiths hosted the rehearsal dinner at home with Betty outdoing herself with the meal preparation, as usual. The wedding was elegant and went without a hitch. Except when it came time to take the official family photograph, Francis went missing. He was somewhere else in the building, exploring all the nooks and crannies as he liked to do, and he completely zoned out that perhaps he was needed for the family photo. So, to this day, a wonderful photograph of the wedding sits in the living room of the Smiths' house—sans Francis.

Senior Year

Before Francis knew it, his whirlwind action-packed summer of 1993 came to a screeching halt. With barely any time to catch his breath, or so it seemed, he was embracing his final senior year at Canterbury High. The workload increased hugely, but much to his delight, it was all in his personal scope of what he considered to be very interesting.

As an alternative to a fourth year of French, Russian was offered. Miss Alla Patterson was a visiting teacher from Moscow, and adding to his interest was the fact that she was particularly attractive. Miss Patterson immediately assigned Russian names to her students. Francis became "Anton." The first order of business was to learn the Cyrillic alphabet. From there, the class studied the vocabulary and conversational language, but most importantly, the students learned grammar and sentence structure. To no one's surprise, Anton or Francis and Miss Patterson developed a close friendship. Learning of his musical talents, she asked him to play Rachmaninoff's *Russian Concerto* for her on the piano. As a thank-you gift, she gave Anton a book of Pushkin's poetry, in Russian, of course, and a few Soviet pins proclaiming Perestroika and Glasnost. During one parent-teacher conference, she told Bob and

Betty their son spoke Russian as if he was a native. At the senior awards ceremony at end of the year, Anton received the school's only Russian prize commendation from Miss Patterson for his excellent work in her class. He dearly loved the language along with anything about the Russian people and culture he could learn. It was very disappointing that, after he graduated, there were no Russian people or resources accessible where he could continue with his newfound passion. Although he can still read the Russian language, sadly his ability to speak it has dwindled away.

The Mad Dentist

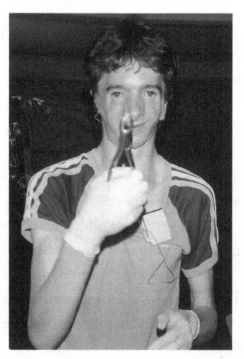

Francis, the Mad Dentist, proudly displays
the tooth he just pulled.

There were other classes Francis was required to take. His two least liked subjects, trigonometry and precalculus, were fortunately taught by Mr. Rieger, a teacher he happened to like very much. Seniors were required to take ethics, which was taught by Mr. DeSalvo; advanced placement (AP) English was taught by Mr. Callicutt, and Mr. Stanley taught U.S. history. Francis's AP history exam score at the end of the year enabled him to completely test out of college history.

Surprisingly, Francis also opted for a second year in jazz band. This time though and much to his relief, he played the grand piano (the instrument he learned on) in place of the keyboard. Jazz taught him to play with gusto, something that his other favored music—classical and sacred music—did not. From those days onward, jazz became a "soundtrack" for his life. He loved the performances, and Bob and Betty were equally enthralled to see such musical enthusiasm from their son. His teacher, Mrs. Kelsey, furthered his interest when she introduced him to jazz and blues piano that became an added musical staple in his life from that point on.

A Miraculous Surprise

Shortly before Christmas of that year and during morning chapel, the students heard a presentation from the Spanish teacher, Dr. Griffin. He spoke of an opportunity for interested students to take an escorted tour of Spain that coming spring. With great animation, he described the historical sites and the itinerary of the "Golden Age of Spain" tour that was offered by Educational Forum, a travel organization that ran student tours all over the world. After chapel, one of the teachers approached Francis and asked him if he was going. Francis replied that he was not because he would only be able to take a trip like that once he became a doctor, the profession he now had his heart set on.

A few weeks later during dinner, the phone rang. Bob got up and answered the phone. No one at the dinner table gave the ongoing conversation much thought until Bob returned to the dinner table with a big smile on his face. Without preamble, he asked his son if he would like to go to Spain. Speechless, Francis managed to at least nod his head yes. Apparently, some anonymous person in the Canterbury School community loved Francis enough to offer to pay his whole way to Spain during spring break. This mystery person somehow managed to secretly set the tour plans in motion, and eventually, his reservation was confirmed for the tour from March 26 to April 4, 1994. The chaperones would be Dr. Griffin himself along with Mrs. Klink whose two daughters, Kristen and Kendra, were taking the trip and a female friend of Dr. Griffin from South America.

Francis could barely contain himself; he was so excited! The days up to the departure day crawled by at a snail's pace in spite of everything he had to get ready for the big day. At last, departure day arrived. Bob drove Francis and Dr. Griffin's friend, the gorgeous Fabiola Aviles from

South America, down from Fort Wayne to Indianapolis. She and Francis had already hit it off, and there were no doubts they were going to be fabulous travel companions. At the Indianapolis airport, they met up with Dr. Griffin and Mrs. Klink and the rest of their entourage. Much to his deep delight, Francis discovered he was the only male student on a trip that was filled with lovely ladies. The entire group boarded the TWA jet, bound for New York City's JFK International Airport to connect with the transatlantic flight to Madrid, Spain. What no one else knew was, in that moment, his childhood dream to someday fly on a Boeing 747 was being fulfilled. He was going to fly on a TWA 747, transatlantic, complete with meals and a movie, no less. He couldn't wait. Just as he settled into his seat, his hearing aid suddenly died, leaving Francis deaf for the entire trip!

Francis soon learned that travel was not for the fainthearted. Upon their arrival in Madrid, the group checked into their hotel then hit the ground running. Not being able to hear was a nuisance, but he wasn't about to allow such a minor detail derail his excitement. Not being able to hear, however, caused a near catastrophe. While crossing a busy street, Francis had gotten separated from the group, and they got ahead of him. Unable to hear the rushing traffic, he attempted to run across the busy road. The rest of the group stood on the other side, watching him with their mouths open, screaming at him to go back. Regardless, unable to hear them, he plunged forward. Cars swerved, brakes squealed, drivers hung out their windows yelling and waving their fists, and his friends screamed. He had nearly caused more than one accident as he made it to the other side. After that, he was never left alone while crossing streets.

The catastrophes didn't stop there. While eating lunch in a restaurant, Francis began to choke on a piece of stringy chicken. Near panic ensued until finally he was able to cough it up. Within the first two hours of being in Madrid, he had almost died twice. From that point on, extra care was taken to keep tabs on him and to not rush him through meals. Not wanting to dwell on the negative, the group made their necessary internal adjustment to meet his needs; then they got right back down to business, visiting the Palacio Real and other historical sites in Madrid.

The next seven days were action-packed. After all, they could rest when they got home. The group traveled around Spain by motor coach, making stops along the way in Toledo, Seville, Cordoba, and Granada, before taking an overnight sleeper train back to Madrid. Despite his hearing loss, he still enjoyed the food, sights, sounds, and the Mediterranean atmosphere of Spain. He shot roll after roll of film that later on would fill up an entire photo album. A pleasant surprise for Francis was that his group deemed him their official mascot, affectionately named "Paco."

This very special trip was the first of many more to come in his future and the one that gave him his love for international travel. To this day, it still remains a secret as to who the mysterious anonymous donor was who gave him this opportunity of a lifetime. This was an unforgettable graduation gift, and to this day, Francis regularly asks in prayer that this wonderful person, or persons, be especially blessed. He is eternally grateful for that wonderful experience.

A Dream in the Making

By now, Francis knew he wanted a career in medicine, specifically as a craniofacial surgeon. The call had come to him during his junior year, but now that he was close to graduating, he was certain of it. For the seniors, it was required that they spend forty hours of their May term as a senior intern in their chosen career field. Since he was well-known and a frequent patient at Riley Hospital and because he knew so many of the doctors and health care professionals there, he approached them about allowing him to intern at the hospital, and they agreed. Canterbury School also agreed to the proposed plan. The long drive was prohibitive, so his friend Trish hosted him in her home with the understanding that he would go back to Fort Wayne on weekends.

For three weeks, Francis followed Dr. Nelson and his colleagues in the operating room as they repaired all manner of facial deformities in children, ranging from cleft palates to skull vault procedures to an all-day long lower jaw procedure similar to what he had undergone before Christmas in 1991. Dr. Nelson challenged Francis that if he could name every instrument on the stands around the operating table, he would receive an A.

Other doctors in the clinic got onboard with Francis's internship, and he was allowed in the clinic and to go along on the ward rounds as they examined children with a diversity of facial anomalies, both outpatient and inpatient. Francis was even allowed to sit in on at least one case conference with the doctors.

In Riley's basement audiology/ENT clinic, Francis's audiologist and her colleagues invited him to be in on hearing tests, speech evaluation, and other ENT procedures. The internship also presented Francis with the opportunity to observe some laboratory research. One medical school student allowed him to sit in while he performed vascular research on mice in his professor's lab. Trish allowed him to help her in the office, and other staff invited him to help with keeping everything organized. What he found most fascinating though was when Dr. Nelson taught him how to make a simple incision and a suture on a pig's foot he got from the supermarket. Francis was over the moon during his internship, and the experience cemented his desire to practice medicine, particularly in craniofacial anomalies. Knowing exactly what he wanted to do with his life inspired him in all things as he moved forward. To this day, he considers this to have been the most valuable experience of his life.

Wedding Bells

Upon arriving back home on a complete high after his three-week internship, Francis was forced back to reality, albeit a happy reality. Christopher was to be married to a tall and beautiful African American woman who lived in Fort

Wayne. The couple had decided to wed in the Smiths' spacious home, so the space was set up for both the rehearsal dinner and the wedding.

Christopher's bride was beautiful in her long lavender gown. There were tears in everyone's eyes as she made her way up to the altar where she met her nervous handsome groom and their pastor, Bob Siegrist. The ceremony was simple yet elegant. At the conclusion, Francis played the recessional—flawlessly, of course.

At the conclusion of the day, the new husband and wife walked out the front door to their car that was festooned with ribbons and "Just Married" signs. The wedding and the shared happiness was a stunning end to a beautiful spring.

The Graduate

Graduation was now only a few weeks away on June 12, 1994. Francis's years at Canterbury High were coming to an end, all too quickly.

On his momentous occasion, almost the entire Smith family attended, arriving in the large white family van. Unlike other schools that wear caps and gowns, the Canterbury High School graduation attire for young men was blue blazers, gray trousers, white shirts, and the official Canterbury school tie; and for the girls, it was a white dress.

Before commencement, the graduates met for the last time in the auditorium where the baccalaureate service was held. Dr. Griffin—the Spanish teacher who was also a brilliant organist—played *Holy, Holy, Holy* as the graduates and families sang along. At the conclusion of this very private service, the graduates marched out the door to the outdoor ceremony. Preceding the procession was a troupe of bag-pipers that played *Amazing Grace*. All the high school students marched behind the graduates in descending order of their grade. It was school tradition that graduation was an affair for everyone to participate in, including the other high school students' families. A stage had been set up outdoors among the trees, and the evening sun shone brightly. The speakers were the headmaster, Mr. Hancock, along with the valedictorian, and a special speaker from the Canterbury community. As each name was called, the graduate approached the podium where they would receive their diploma in that one special moment that was theirs alone.

Years later, Francis was fascinated to learn on his own that all of Canterbury School's traditions were borrowed from English schools, and Canterbury had gotten its name and crest from England's Canterbury Cathedral.

After what seemed like an eternity, Francis's name was called. A great cheer rang out from the audience, including the graduates on stage. If ever there was a moment of crowning glory for him and his family, this moment was it. Graduation was an incredible milestone and achievement for any high school student, but for someone who was as challenged—including emotionally challenged—as he was, it is the one moment in his life that stands out above all others. It was at Canterbury High School that Francis was able to truly heal from the bullying that had left such a deep fear and hurt no one thought he would be able to move forward. The scar was still there, but it was now covered with a thicker hide and a level of compassion for others who suffered as he had. His experience at Canterbury—with the teachers, staff, and his peers—was a monumental one that gave him back his love of life, music, medicine, and a restored faith in humanity. This was a wonderful moment.

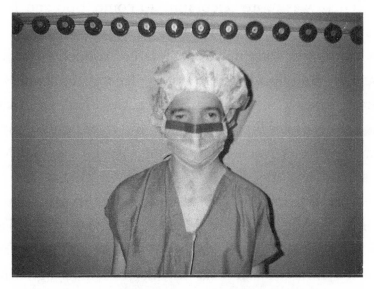

During Francis's senior year medical internship, he was more certain than ever that he wanted a career in medicine.

After much celebration, it was time to say goodbye. The moment was incredibly heartfelt and bittersweet. Seemingly, it took forever to say goodbye to his personal angel, Elizabeth, Mr. and Mrs. Hancock, his teachers, his peers, and close personal friends; but he didn't want to miss anyone who had played a part in the most amazing four years of his life. There were tears, hugs, and promises to remain in touch.

Bob finally gave the signal that it was time to move on. Destination: ice cream! The entire family gathered around several tables at Atz's Ice Cream, a Fort Wayne icon and a family favorite, to celebrate this momentous occasion. Finally, it was time to leave and head home and to bed.

There was more celebrating to come. Bob and Betty and Francis's siblings planned for a graduation open house at their home, out on the very large wooden deck. For hours, it was a nonstop procession of extended family and friends from school, church, and many others from various phases of his life. The pastors and their families came. His Canterbury teachers: Mr. King, Mr. Furiak, and Mrs. Sessions—his "Big Three"—came to celebrate. But the most heartwarming of all was the arrival of many family friends from his distant childhood years such as his piano teacher Mrs. Kelsey, the Matzes, Wilhelms, and other families they knew. Some dear friends from long ago when Francis first became a part of the Smith family, including Myra Conley, his first speech therapist, arrived. What a memorable joyous day this was!

Commit your works to the Lord
And your plans will be established.
—Proverbs 16:3

The Canterbury High School graduate.

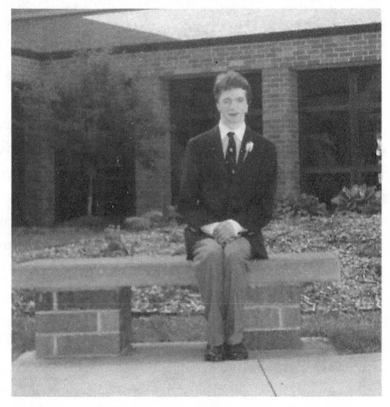

A memorable day, a day of personal achievement,
healing, and strong sense of direction.

A Movie Star Named Cher

In 1985, pop-star-turned-movie-star Cher starred in
the film *Mask*, depicting the true story of Rocky Dennis,
masterfully played by Eric Stoltz, who suffered from the
craniofacial deformity, craniodiaphyseal dysplasia, nicknamed "lionitis," a disease that eventually claimed his life.
This outstanding memorable film touched on Rocky's

struggle to find acceptance in the public school system where "looks and popularity" were paramount while dealing with the fact that his life expectancy was short. Eventually, Rocky found acceptance in the biker crowd of his mother, Rusty (powerfully played by Cher). While battling her own demons—drug, alcohol, and sex addiction—Rusty proved to be a ruthless advocate for her son. Although this bittersweet film sadly ends with Rocky's death, it's his victory of winning the respect and friendships of his high school peers and even finding true love that carries this film. Cher was so profoundly affected by Rocky's true story she became the celebrity national spokeswoman for the Children's Craniofacial Association (CCA).

The summer of his graduation, 1994, Francis attended his first craniofacial family retreat, run by the CCA, in Indianapolis. Bob, Betty, Francis, Ruth, and Courtney, James's daughter, went down for the weekend. It was an exciting time to meet other families with children who had facial differences and were able to share their life stories with others. The disorders ranged from cleft lip and palate to very rare and sometimes severe syndromes, such as Treacher Collins syndrome, Goldenhar, Apert, and Crouzon syndromes. There were also other adults who were afflicted who came along. At the retreat, Francis made a goodly number of friends whom he would subsequently meet at other CCA retreats for years to come.

Trish Severns from Riley Hospital for Children was there, and she arranged for Francis to play something on the piano for everyone there. In the hotel ballroom, Francis played the second movement, "Adagio" from Beethoven's *Sonata Pathetique, Op. 13*, on the grand piano. From that point on, it became tradition for Francis to perform at the retreats. On behalf of the doctors at Riley Clinic A, Trish presented him with a copy of *Dorland's Illustrated Medical Dictionary*, signed by his doctors at Riley, as a graduation gift.

CCA would become a staple in Francis's life as it would with many of the friends he met through the group. Cher actually became more than just a passing acquaintance, and he has many photographic mementos of the group and even of several personal meetings over the years with Cher herself.

***

Before the summer was over, Rob, the other twin, got married. Rob met his beloved while he was working at a homeless shelter. The two fell in love and married at the Garrett United Methodist Church. Even though everyone, by now, were old hands at weddings, their union was still met with great excitement, and once again, another family wedding unfolded beautifully.

The summer of 1994 was an exciting one, but most of all, it became the setting for the next major setting in Francis's life: college!

Ruth, Cher, Francis

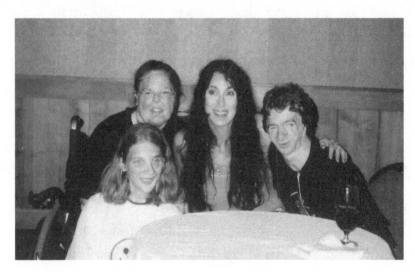

"Cher is all heart," says Francis.

Book 4

That you may not grieve as others do
who have no hope...

—1 Thessalonians 4:13

Chapter 1

An Unexpected Farewell
1995

Turning Point

With enormous gratitude toward some very special friends the LORD used between his sophomore and junior years to convince him that he could best serve others by having a career in medicine, Francis was already focused on a biology major. That decision led him toward a specific specialty, that of craniofacial surgery. So, for his junior and senior years at Canterbury High, he focused on a premedical university education. Canterbury has always had a very high college acceptance rate, with over 90 percent of its students continuing on to major state or private universities, not to mention Ivy League and other prestigious colleges.

Late into his junior year, Francis decided to apply to Indiana University-Purdue University Fort Wayne (IPFW), which is a local satellite campus of both Indiana University and Purdue University. This choice was logical because the campus was close to home, and it also provided a high-quality biology premed curriculum from the well-known Purdue University. He felt confident that he probably could have gone on to a bigger state or even Ivy League university had it not been for the high expense. Attached to his application were the results of the required SAT and ACT tests. Barely one year later during his senior year, he learned he had been accepted into the Purdue Bachelor of Science in Biology program. Several scholarships that he had won by his academic merit and life experiences were ready.

In the spring of 1994, not long before his high school graduation, Francis was invited to interview by the head of the biology department on the Purdue campus. The office of Dr. Richard Manalis was located in the basement of Kettler Hall, the sixties vintage main building where the biology department was housed at that time. Bob, Betty, and Francis were warmly and enthusiastically welcomed into his office that was cluttered to capacity with his journals, books, physiological measuring equipment, and all the other equipment that mark the life of a busy biology professor. The professor listened attentively as he watched an animated Francis regale him with his life story and educational prowess at Canterbury. At the end, Dr. Manalis introduced Francis to the requirements of the biology curriculum and its electives. Another wonderful relationship with a strong rapport was formed.

Francis visited the IPFW campus several times that summer in order for more discussions with future faculty about the program as well as for student orientation, advising, and registration (SOAR). Scores of new freshmen converged on the campus to attend introductory talks by university officials, campus tours, and, most importantly, one-on-one advising for their individual freshman year curricula. Along with biology and physiology, he registered for chemistry, a class he previously struggled with. French, English composition, finite mathematics, and several other courses rounded out seventeen credit hours, which was more than a full load.

Making Changes

Francis's freshman year workload looked pretty heavy on paper. The reality was it was far worse.

Routine all-nighters, fueled by a near–Mountain Dew addiction, consistently left Francis with little-to-no sleep and the accompanying nausea many college students experience. He sucked it up and kept moving forward even against the protestations of his parents. He and Ruth were the only two children at home now, so at least the atmosphere was no longer hectic. It was almost too calm.

What Betty was keeping to herself was Bob's health was steadily declining. That Thanksgiving in 1994, Bob had to be taken to Lutheran Hospital in Fort Wayne where he spent several weeks in the coronary ICU, hooked up to a respirator. He wasn't allowed to come home until right before Christmas.

For years, Betty begged her husband to quit smoking, but like millions of other smokers, he was addicted. His numerous attempts to acquiesce to his wife's pleadings failed time and time again, and now his health was irretrievably on a downward death spiral. Bob was under almost constant medical care as his emphysema worsened. Life went on as normally as possible so as not to upset Francis and Ruth, but they couldn't help but notice that their father was constantly out of breath and could barely live his life anymore. Bob always drove Francis to college and back again, and even that was becoming a difficult chore.

Now that Francis was in college, he decided it was time that he learn how to drive. Due to his hearing and visual impairments, he was referred to a driving school in Fort Wayne for people with disabilities called Safeway Driving School. On Christmas Eve, an evaluator from Safeway came to the Smiths' home in a black Dodge Neon. Francis was so excited he practically jumped behind the wheel. With the evaluator riding shotgun, he began driving around the neighborhood. Not surprisingly, he took to it naturally.

After their initial drive, a Safeway instructor came to the IPFW on a regular basis for Francis's instruction. In no time at all, they were driving all over the big city of Fort Wayne. Like any driver's education vehicle, it was equipped with a brake on the passenger side that his instructor used on a number of different occasions to keep him from getting into some precariously close calls. That said, Francis acclimated to city driving quite quickly. From there, he graduated to highway driving on the Interstate 69 freeway that ran past Fort Wayne.

Bob wasted no time taking his son out driving while he rode shotgun. Every now and then, Bob let loose with some unbecoming language when Francis flew over a railroad-crossing grade or made a mad sudden turn or came to a brake-slamming stop. It was a family tradition that whenever Bob taught one of his children to drive and they "almost killed" him in a near accident, he would take them to the local Penguin Point fast-food restaurant to thank them for not killing him. With Francis though, that never became a necessity. The hard work paid off. Just before his twentieth birthday in April 1995, Francis took his driving test in New Haven and earned his driver's license. Right before the test, his instructor turned to him and asked him if he believed in prayer, which of course he did.

To celebrate this newest milestone, Francis went to the Crisis Pregnancy Center where Betty volunteered once a week to show her his new license. She was thrilled.

The Smith family's blue 1986 Chevrolet Cavalier station wagon was now his to drive to and from campus. Francis complied by paying for the gas and the insurance. He loved station wagons, and he considered this to be his "first" car although it would be two decades before he actually purchased a station wagon out of his own money.

Even though the driving load was lifted from Bob, his health was rapidly declining. He now suffered from congestive heart failure along with his emphysema and was pretty much housebound and on oxygen. When Francis was home from school, he spent quite a bit of time helping with his father's oxygen cannula and tanks. But during his freshman year, his father's health nose-dived. In May, Bob and Betty discussed with the doctors about a procedure called "cardioversion," a critical surgery where the heart would be stopped then shocked back into a normal rhythm.

After that discussion, Betty took Bob to see his doctor for a follow-up appointment. While examining him, the doctor put down his stethoscope and shook his head. He told Bob to go home. No other words were spoken.

That moment still haunts Betty to this day.

A New Arrival in Heaven

A few days later, Betty and her husband knelt by the side of their marital bed in prayer, as they had done every night of their marriage when they were home together. Slowly, methodically, he prayed for each of their children by name, asking for their LORD's guidance and protection in each of their lives. Instead of coming to bed with Betty, he said he was going to the bathroom, which was a shared bathroom down the hall. Betty turned out the lights and put her head on the pillow. She fell fast asleep.

In the early hours of May 31, Betty awoke with a start. Turning over, she discovered the bed was empty.

When Betty opened the door to the hallway, she could see that the bathroom light was on. She put on her robe and padded down the hallway. She knocked on the bathroom door. It opened slightly. The bathroom was empty.

Across the hall was a spare bedroom. The door was partially closed. Softly, she called Bob's name. There was no answer. The moon shone through the bedroom window, and in silhouette, she could see her husband sitting on the end of the bed. Relieved, she walked over and gently touched him on the shoulder. The soft touch was enough to make him fall backward onto the bed. On his face was a look of peace. He was gone.

Betty cradled her dead husband in her arms before releasing him. She went down the hallway, waking Francis and Ruth. Together, the three of them went back to the spare bedroom where Bob lay on top of the bed. There is no memory as to who called 911. They held hands, cried, and prayed as the sirens of the approaching first responders got closer and closer to the house.

Apparently, Bob suspected his time to go home was near. They all believed he moved to the guest bedroom in order to spare Betty the trauma of finding her husband gone in their bed. EMTs, firefighters, and police crowded into the house. Heroically, the EMTs tried to revive him even as his body was placed inside the ambulance. Betty, Francis, and Ruth followed the ambulance to DeKalb Memorial Hospital. Susie and her husband were already at the hospital by the time they arrived.

They clung tightly together until the doctor came out to tell them that despite everything they could do to try to revive him, they could not. They were then allowed into the trauma bay where Bob lay, looking so peaceful. Betty knew at once where her husband really was.

Absent from the body, present with the LORD.

—2 Corinthians 5:8

There would be no more pain, no more gasping for breath. Together, they stood, holding one another, each of them hit hard by their loss, each coping with Bob's death in their own special way. They cried and prayed and bid him farewell. Bob was Betty's husband for over forty years and their father.

A Massive Void

Later, slightly before dawn when they returned home, there was a peculiar emptiness about it. Where Bob's earthly life had once filled their home with his presence, there was now a strange empty void. Francis became physically ill from the shock. Due to his autism, it was rare for him to ever show emotion, and for the first time that he can ever remember, he actually shed tears. His father's death wasn't a complete surprise by any stretch of the imagination, but when it happened, it was surreal.

Word spread quickly. While it was still quite early in the morning, the house began to fill with family and friends. Their pastor arrived, followed by several other members of the church. As morning transitioned into early noon, the house was filled with even more friends, many bringing food. That day was a heartbreaking one that was filled with shock, tears, and disbelief, punctuated with sudden jolts of tearful reality.

None of the family could afford to wallow in their grief for long. There was too much to do. Betty and Edwin went to the funeral home in Auburn to make the funeral arrangements for Bob's services. Betty had asked Angel to give the eulogy for their father, and she agreed, on the spot.

It just so happened that Susie was also going to give a speech at the DeKalb High School baccalaureate service that night. Bob, Betty, and several other children had planned to be there to hear her speak. In their shock and grief, it was decided that the family would still attend to support Susie. From the podium with hundreds of eyes upon her, Susie flawlessly eulogized her amazing father to the students, their families, and friends. There wasn't a dry eye among them. In spite of her grief, Betty heard each and every loving testimonial word.

On Friday, June 2, the Smiths spent the evening at Bob's wake at the funeral home, receiving so many who had come to pay their respects. The chapel was filled with countless people they knew and countless more they did not but whose lives had been touched in some way by Bob's example. Mom insisted that he be prepared for his casket in the casual attire he was known by everyone to wear—comfortable, not stuffy. His white shirtsleeves were rolled up; his floral-print tie was loose, and he wore matching floral-print suspenders and no jacket. The oak casket was covered in red roses and ribbons. Bouquets that were given by Magnavox, the church, and even Riley Hospital surrounded the casket. James's five-year-old daughter and Francis's niece, Courtney, asked Francis why her grandpa was lying in a crib, a gesture so reminiscent of when his older brother Peter had died, and he had asked nearly the same question to his sister Angel. Young children who have never seen a casket and can't quite grasp death have an amazing coping mechanism to help them try to understand the unimaginable. To Francis, Peter's casket had been the "dying trunk."

***

The night before Bob's funeral and interment, Betty fell into a fitful sleep. In the middle of the night, Ruth awakened her to tell her someone was at the door. She put on her bathrobe and slippers and padded down the hall, then down the stairs to the front door. Looking through the peephole, she saw a figure standing under the porch light, shrouded in a khaki-colored raincoat. The hood obscured his face. Betty answered the door.

"Yes?" she said.

The hooded figure didn't say anything. In his hand was a triangular package. He handed it to Betty, then turned, and left.

Betty brought the package in and placed it on the dining room table. Ruth was there. She handed her mother a pair of scissors. Slowly, Betty opened the brown paper packaging. Inside was a perfectly folded American flag. On top of it was a note card with "Dad" written on top in eerily familiar handwriting.

"Andrew."

Betty woke and bolted upright, her heart pounding, with sweat on her forehead. She turned on the light, and no one was there. For the rest of the night, she tossed and turned. There was no more sleep.

Bob Must Be Camping in Heaven

Heaven cried an abundance of tears on that very sad day of Bob's funeral and burial. Being a musical family, a great deal of thought was put into choosing the music everyone knew Bob would love, and his children chose his music accordingly. Francis accompanied his sister Angel on the piano while she sang "The LORD's Prayer." Christopher sang one of his father's favorites, *On Eagle's Wings*. Rob read aloud from the children's book, *The Giving Tree*. He often said that his father was so much like the tree that gave all it had. Susie gave a repeat more in-depth version of the wonderful eulogy she gave for her father at DeKalb High School.

When Bob passed away, someone called the prison where James was incarcerated to let him know his father had died. On the day of the funeral, a Department of Corrections van brought a heartbroken James to the church so he could see his father one last time. Bob had been the center of his life, the only dad he had ever known ever known, and he loved him through and through. He was heartbroken.

Fighting the torrential downpour, the pallbearers lifted their father's casket from the hearse and, once again, struggled under its great weight to get it to the gravesite. The rain was relentless. Francis took his place next to Betty. In a moment of humor, Betty leaned over and whispered to him, "This is just like camping."

Chapter 2

God at Work in Their Lives

The Three Musketeers

Now that Bob was gone, there was a great deal of shifting and constant adjusting to find for themselves their "new normal." In spite of Betty, Francis, and Ruth's great heartbreak and sadness, they kept moving forward, one step, one day at a time, all the while clinging mightily to the LORD for comfort and direction. After all, the LORD was always doing mighty work in their lives, even in their great sorrow. What often kept them moving forward when all they really wanted to do was sink into sadness was they knew this was what Bob would have wanted. He never would have tolerated anything less. In Betty's words, they were the "Three Musketeers" against the world.

In spite of her deep grief, Betty forged ahead. With Bob's constant travels, she was often left to hold down the fort on her own. This lessened as his illness progressed, but her husband was still the head of the household and the breadwinner, not to mention a hands-on caring dad. Now she had to assume all the responsibilities required to run a home, not to mention she somehow had to come up with an income. What she could do immediately, she did. She sold the RV that Bob had driven every summer for their campouts, and in its place, she bought a tent so they could continue camping. The large white van was traded for a smaller more manageable Dodge minivan. Ruth, who had been homeschooled for several years, now needed to be enrolled in school. Thankfully, Betty's brother Bob stepped up to the plate and paid for one year of her tuition so she could go back to school. True to His word, the LORD never failed to provide for any of their needs.

A Nasty Infection

That summer, the Three Musketeers flew to Boston to attend their second CCA retreat. At Chicago O'Hare airport, they met up with an older couple they had met at the Indianapolis retreat the year before, and their friendship picked up again as if no time in between had passed. To Francis, they were all simply "family." Per his new tradition, Francis played the piano for the crowd in the ballroom where everyone gathered for fun and games. Some of the group went out on a lobster boat in the Boston harbor. The next day, several members of the group visited Plymouth Plantation where costumed actors recreated the lives of the pilgrims and their American Indian companions. From there, they traveled on to Plymouth Rock where the group boarded a replica of The Mayflower II, complete with actors who portrayed sailors and passengers. On the last day of the gathering, they walked a short distance on the Freedom Trail and visited the Old North Church.

What Francis failed to mention to anyone was one of his implants was infected again. For Francis, they returned home to Fort Wayne just in time. On the flight home, the pain, then swelling, became almost unendurable in the pressurized cabin. Betty wasted no time in getting him straight to Riley Hospital where some of the fluid was removed with a syringe to test it for bacteria. With an infection verified, Francis was scheduled for surgery to drain and irrigate the infected site. Francis spent the next week in the hospital with strong antibiotics being fed through an IV. Once again, his veins began to collapse, so they had to reinsert the IV in the emergency room.

Two Lovely Journalists

In the fall of 1995, Francis returned to IPFW as a sophomore. Since he had failed finite mathematics the previous year, he was required to retake that class, this time with a tutor. He found the one-on-one help to be immensely helpful, and this time, he passed the class with a B. Organic chemistry replaced general chemistry, and he found organic chemistry more palatable. But his favorite course was on communication disorders that focused on speech and language disorders. Because of his own life experiences with cleft palate speech, he was actually able to lecture the class about his speech disorder and craniofacial anomalies.

***

One evening right after dinner, two lovely women from the Fort Wayne newspaper *The News Sentinel* arrived unannounced at the house. Someone from the university must have talked to the paper because these two women were there to prepare a feature story on Francis. Over the course of several weeks, they came for several hours at a time where they interviewed Betty, Francis, and several other members of the family and close friends about his struggle with Treacher Collins syndrome. They photographed him studying at his desk in his room and reveled in his "medical and surgical museum" where he had collected years' worth of the medical artifacts associated with his medical care and numerous surgeries. This included his feeding syringes, craniofacial implants and facial space fillers, wires that held his jaws together, etc. The ladies were duly impressed! This was a great kickoff to his dreams and ambitions of entering medicine as a career, perhaps as a craniofacial surgeon. The ladies even attended church with the Smiths twice and followed him around campus where they actually sat in on two of his courses.

The end result of the hard work of these two inquisitive reporters resulted in an admirable and revealing feature story of Francis's life that unfolded in the November

4, 1995 *News Sentinel.* The layout covered several pages complete with photographs. To see his life encapsulated in print, complete with images, was a penetrating experience. There were no more uncomfortable stares when he passed by someone who didn't know how to react to his physical appearance. In their place were looks of admiration.

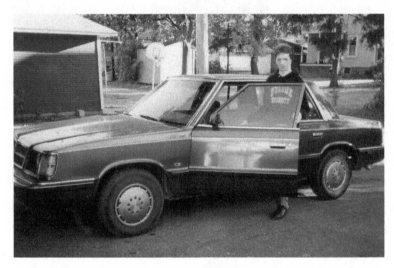

Francis's first car: 1989 Dodge Aries K sedan.

Back on the Nonstop

Francis still had to face the reality that his struggles were far from over. The below-the-eye implant was subject to recurring infections that required immediate medical care. The infections were so frequent they resulted in the doctors making the decision to remove the implant.

Meanwhile, in the spring of 1996, Francis continued with organic chemistry and statistics. Molecular genetics was the subject he was the most fascinated by because he had recently heard about the discovery of the gene for Treacher Collins syndrome in the early nineties by Dr. Dixon at the University of Manchester in Manchester, England. This breakthrough event is what sparked his interest in genetics while he was still in high school. He also improved his analytical writing skills in an expository writing course.

That summer, Francis got his first job as a carryout person in Scott's Foods grocery store in Auburn. He easily made friends with his boss, coworkers, and customers; and he loved it. With faithful diligence, he saved his money, and before too long, he was able to buy his first car. It was a very big day when Betty and Francis arrived at Sanderson's Used Car Lot along the Auburn strip. Together, they looked over several suitable cars before he settled on a twilight blue 1989 Dodge Aries K sedan. It looked almost showroom new, most likely because its only previous owner had been an elderly lady who lived in the area, and she only drove it on short errands. After the salesman took them on a test drive, the deal was sealed. Francis was so proud of his "new baby," and no one who crossed his path got away without the requisite *oooohs* and *aaaahs*.

***

Time seemed to travel by at warp speed, and before they knew it, it was time for another CCA family retreat, this time in Chicago, which was close enough to drive to. Gathering a few friends along the way whom they had met the previous year at the Boston CCA, the time passed by quickly.

The CCA event took place at the grand old Palmer House Hilton in the Loop where Francis didn't waste any time setting himself down at the piano to serenade old and new friends alike. During a Cubs game the group attended at Wrigley Field against the Cincinnati Reds (who beat the Cubs), Francis scored an autographed baseball from Jaime Navarro, a souvenir that remains with him to this day. Ruth one-upped him by getting hers from legendary Cubs announcer Hary Caray himself. The retreat ended with a visit to the Museum of Science and Industry, a favorite haunt of the Smiths over the Christmas holidays in years past.

***

The 1996–1997 school year at Purdue was unlike any other. Francis definitely showed a strong desire for anything science and medicine. It appeared that just about every course he took was science or medical oriented. In microbiology, he grew colonies of different species of bacteria in petri dishes, and once, he had to identify an unknown species using a battery of experiments. In cellular neurophysiology, he studied the structure of nerve cells and how electrical impulses travel from one nerve cell to the next along a nerve. He also took physics and child psychology. From there, he went on to physics and calculus, earning all As, plus an intensive course in animal physiology, with an attached lab class in which he covered topics ranging from nerve impulse transmission to digestion and waste filtering to circulation. What turned out to be his favorite class though was abnormal psychology.

In the summer of 1997, Francis was invited to participate in a physiological research experiment with Dr. Manalis, his physiology professor and academic mentor. While Dr. Manalis and several other students did the experiments, Francis did extensive research, looking for recent pertinent articles on transport of molecules through red blood cell membranes through a process of facilitated diffusion through channels in the membrane, which is an all-important research in the field of medicine. He kept them abreast of his findings.

A Defining Event

In the summer of 1997, Francis learned that his hero, Dr. Dixon, was coming to New York City in July to give the keynote lecture at a Treacher Collins syndrome symposium. Francis's longtime dream was to someday meet Dr. Dixon, and nothing, not even Betty's protestations for his safety and concerns about him traveling alone, was going to hold him back from being there. While making his travel arrangements, he planned on spending an extra day in New York for sightseeing.

On Saturday evening, he arrived and checked into a clean, more-than-adequate hotel on Thirty-fourth Street, not far from the Empire State Building. Sunday morning, Francis wasted no time getting on the subway to JFK International Airport for no other purpose than to engage in plane spotting and to visit several of the architecturally unique airline terminals. The one that fascinated him the most was the otherworldly main building of the TWA terminal with its flowing concrete that somewhat resembled a bird that graduated into a guitar-shaped concourse. Designed by Eero Saarinen, this was the very terminal from where he and several of his high school friends departed from on their way to Spain several years prior, which evoked so many fond memories. Happily ensconced in this wonderful world of design, he had to push himself to move on. After spending some time watching planes take off and land, he went off to visit some of the other unique terminals at JFK.

Finally, he headed back to Manhattan where he visited the World Trade Center. From the cavernous, cathedral-like lobby of the Twin Towers, he boarded the rapid elevator ride to the Observation Deck on the one hundred seventh floor where he spent over an hour looking over the entire city and the surrounding miles. For dinner, he treated himself at Sbarro's Italian Eatery located on the deck where afterward he had his photo taken in a photo booth. With some money he had saved, he bought a bronze cast replica of the Twin Towers. Just before he boarded the rapid elevator to take him back to the lobby of the Twin Towers, he stopped and turned back around, and for the next few moments, he surveyed every inch of the Observation Deck. In that moment, he didn't want to leave; he wanted a firm memory of this time etched into his memory forever. After all, he had no way of knowing when, or if, he would ever come back here, and he wanted to remember every single detail he could about the very special time he was able to spend there.

Next, Francis trekked back toward the Empire State Building. From its gorgeous Art Deco lobby, he boarded the fast elevator to the eighty-sixth floor where he stepped out onto the outdoor deck and took in the twilight panorama of the city. For the rest of that evening and well past midnight, he walked all over lower Manhattan, eventually ending up at Times Square. Nothing though was more exciting to him as was the day of the symposium the next day.

On Monday, Francis walked the few short blocks from his hotel to the New York University Medical Center on Thirty-fourth Street. He spent the entire day listening to several speakers talking about the clinical, psychological, and family aspects of raising a child of Treacher Collins syndrome.

Then came the moment Francis had been waiting for. Dr. Dixon gave the keynote speech in which he described his work since the early nineties on the discovery and isolation of the particular gene on chromosome 5 that causes Treacher Collins syndrome when it is mutated. He described the process of how he came to find the gene, then what mutations he found to blame for the syndrome. Francis hung onto and absorbed every word. Afterward, Francis had the opportunity to speak with Dr. Dixon, a conversation that only served to fuel a growing desire for what would eventually become his own life's work. There would be other meetings with. Dr. Dixon in the future.

Back to the Future

When Francis returned to IPFW in the fall of 1997, there was new meaning behind his desire to move forward in the medical field, and he was completely excited. Based on his research project on water transport through red blood cell membranes with Dr. Manalis, he wrote up a minithesis based on his extensive research through recent journal articles on that topic. With great enthusiasm, he pursued a variety of other courses that included archaeology, psychobiology, and the one course he really loved—drawing. Before he knew it, he was in his last school year before graduation.

Now that Francis was a senior, it was mandatory that he facilitate a senior biology seminar to the entire biology department. Since he was following Dr. Dixon's work on the genetics of Treacher Collins syndrome, it was only natural that he chose that topic for his presentation.

Francis put together a detailed presentation that began with the background of the syndrome then progressed into its genetics and pathology. The presentation garnered a great deal of interest in the audience that was composed of students and faculty, all who engaged in his passion for the topic. After the presentation, Francis spent quite a bit of time answering questions.

The spring 1998 semester, however, was nearly derailed. Somewhere along the way, he developed a very painful corneal ulcer on his right eye. In the midst of a heavy workload that consisted of sociology, classical mythology, population ecology, and analytical chemistry, he was fighting against terrible pain. For months, he was treated with antibiotic eye drops and a patch over his right eye that certainly limited his already-challenged vision. The pain was so intense he actually wanted to lose his eye—anything to bring him some prayed-for relief. Finally, slowly, his eye healed.

***

By divine appointment, in May of 1998, Francis ran into a local doctor in Auburn, Dr. Souder, who had a family practice and worked at DeKalb Memorial Hospital. Francis was there for some now-forgotten reason, and the good doctor remembered him. The connection appeared to be that Dr. Souder had a child at Canterbury High School, so he remembered Francis from his graduation. Somehow, he was aware of his burgeoning interest in medicine, and he offered to allow Francis to shadow him so he could learn what it was like to be a doctor. For the entire summer, he spent five days a week in Dr. Souder's office, shadowing him as he consulted with and treated each of his many patients. Dr. Souder made copies of Francis's chapter from the Jill Krementz book *How It Feels to Live with a Physical Disability* and put them in each of the consultation rooms for patients to read if they desired. Many of the patients who read the pages immediately recognized Francis, so there was no lack of conversation when he stood in with the doctor.

What really excited Francis though was being able to accompany Dr. Souder on his rounds at DeKalb Hospital. He had an immediate rapport with the doctor's nursing staff of six nurses and was invited to attend surgical procedures. On surgery days, he gowned up and observed Dr. Souder as he administered general anesthesia.

Dr. Souder's wonderful generosity did not stop there. Before long, Francis was being introduced to his colleagues in Fort Wayne, including a radiologist, surgeons, cardiologists, and others, all who invited him to shadow them. He visited a cancer ward at Lutheran Hospital and the pathology department at Parkview Hospital where he observed an autopsy. He learned quickly that he had nerves of steel for, after the procedure, he ate a full lunch. Next on his busy list was a plastic surgeon that allowed him to stand in while he performed a breast augmentation or reduction, liposuction, and other cosmetic procedures. The more serious surgeries were done in an actual operating room.

The months that Francis graciously spent with Dr. Souder were the most exciting of his life. When he returned to IPFW in the fall of 1998 for the last half of his four and a half years there, he was never more certain that what he wanted to do the most in his life was to become a surgeon that specialized in craniofacial anomalies.

Francis also took advantage of what was probably the last time he would ever have the opportunity to study literature in-depth by studying the world masterpieces that included Dante's *Inferno*, a gruesome fourteenth-century travelogue of the nine descending circles of hell, as well as *Sir Gawain and the Green Knight* and several others. Also included in his studies were the exploration of world folklore and social psychology. Last, he studied structure and pathology of viruses in the virology course, culminating in his achieving his coveted bachelor of science degree.

College Grad

In May 1999, in the huge nearby Allen County War Memorial Coliseum arena that was packed with graduating students from all departments, as well as faculty, officials, and families, Francis was conferred with his bachelor's degree in biology from Purdue University. Betty, Ruth, Susie, and several other family members were in the audience that evening as were several family friends.

Ruth had also reached a milestone of her own: she had graduated from Lakewood Park Christian School, formerly known as Faith Christian Academy. The next day, the Smiths' home was filled with family and friends of both Francis and Ruth, including their family pastor, some former teachers, and Lee Durland, Betty's nurse friend who helped teach Betty how to care for Francis when he was first brought into the Smiths' home. Francis's cake had the logo of Purdue University on it, and on Ruth's cake were butterflies since butterflies were her favorite motif.

With the excitement over, Francis began the daunting task of applying to medical schools all over the United States, including Indiana University School of Medicine in Indiana whose hospitals included Riley Hospital. So began the very long arduous period of waiting, something Francis admittedly was not very good at. It was a lesson where the LORD taught Francis patience and perseverance.

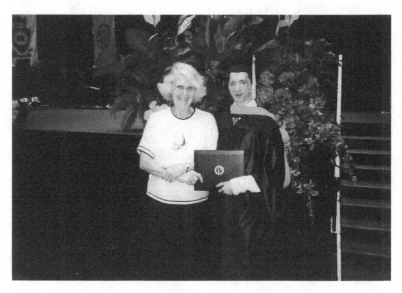

Betty and Francis at his graduation
from Purdue University.

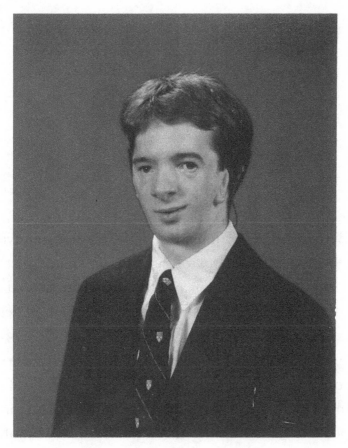

Francis Smith's senior portrait.

Chapter 3

Unwavering Faith
1999–2001

The Graduate Years

Betty's source of inner strength was her unwavering faith in the LORD along with her trust in His perfect timing. Through devoted prayer and her many trials that only served to strengthen these attributes, she longingly desired to pass such faith on to her children.

Francis, for certain, was one child of Betty who had developed his own strong desire to walk with the LORD, but there were times that impatience and frustration got the best of him. Finding the right medical school is a daunting process in and of itself, but when a person is challenged, the chances are even slimmer of getting into the school of their choice. Francis was about to find that out.

"That was a terribly difficult time for Francis when all the rejections came in. They felt he wasn't social enough.

My heart broke for him. But look at him now," remembered Betty.

"Francis thought of himself as a failure because he had so many rejections. A lot of my children felt that way at some point in their journey. It was very difficult for all of them," remembered Betty sadly. "The concern for Francis, specifically, was because of his disabilities, he would not be able to communicate in the way a doctor needs to be able to communicate with their patients." Although it was tough on Betty, she never missed an opportunity to pray for and encourage her son while they patiently endured the waiting game.

Francis had no other choice than to do his part, and that was to go through the process while praying and placing his trust and patience in the LORD to work things out. It was to be a long journey that was inevitably fraught with many disappointments before he was led to the right place, and when that finally happened, it was the best experience he ever could have even hoped for because he knew it came from the LORD. What both Betty and Francis firmly believed was that all of Francis's efforts and achievements would not be wasted. The LORD would use those and all his talents for His purposes. They both had peace, knowing that Francis was on the right track.

Until that time was revealed, Francis pursued every avenue and knocked on every door he possibly could. As part of the process, he took the Medical College Admission Test (MCAT) in the spring of 1999 at Ball State University in Muncie, Indiana. What he remembers is that it was the most unexpectedly difficult test he had ever taken. Aside from hundreds of multiple-choice questions in biology, chemistry, physics, and other sciences, the test dealt with mathematical reasoning and verbal or language arts. The caveat, however, were several critical-thinking essay questions. The test was so long he actually stayed the night before it in a local motel. A month later, he got the results. He hadn't done so well. His score was the devil's number—666!

During that long difficult month of waiting, Francis submitted an application to Indiana University School of Medicine in Indianapolis, of which Riley's Hospital was a part. The American Medical College Admissions Services had a common form that could be filled out and mailed back to them with his desired medical school, Indiana University, listed on it for them to forward to the school itself. Along with this lengthy detailed form, he was required to submit his up-to-date academic transcript from Purdue. After another long period of waiting, he received information from Indiana University requesting supplementary documents from him, including letters of recommendation from professors and others who knew him well. After he responded, he waited, again.

After a wait of several weeks, Francis received an invitation to interview at Indiana University School of Medicine that spring. Since this was to be an all-day event, he traveled to Indianapolis the night before and stayed in a motel near downtown.

The next morning, Francis drove over to the IUPUI/ Indiana University Medical Center campus where he and other prospective students were treated to a guided tour of the medical center campus, including Riley Hospital, which was so familiar to him, and the medical research and teaching buildings.

Francis kept his focus on his dream of becoming a doctor, knowing many people were praying for him. He was not about to give up, and he refused to allow the serious competition he faced to deter him. At one point during the interview, he was advised to get a master's degree in biology to enhance his chances in the program.

Purdue

Taking the advice he was given, Francis applied for the Purdue biology master's degree program at IPFW for entry in the fall of 1999. A short time later, he was notified that he was accepted as a new graduate student in the biology department. As soon as he was able to meet with Dr. Steven Kuhl, the professor he chose to be his academic and research advisor throughout his program, he would be able to plan the curriculum for his next two years. Francis also had to set up a committee of several professors who taught courses in a number of other areas of his interest. These courses included biochemistry, physiology, microbiology, immunology, and molecular genetics. He enjoyed physiology and molecular genetics and most of his other classes, but he struggled the hardest with biochemistry.

A major portion of Francis's master degree requirements was to be a laboratory research project. His major's
professor Dr. Steven Kuhl was a microbiologist who had his
own laboratory. For an entire year, he worked with the bacterium *Bordetella pertussis*, which causes pertussis (whooping
cough). He cultured the nasty bacterium in petri dishes and
introduced specially altered DNA into them. He learned to
isolate and purify the DNA that was in these cells. Soon,
his professor came to call him his "DNA isolation man."
Adding some humor to the stressful course since this was
the turn of the century and the Y2K "computer bug" was
reaching hysteria proportions, Francis privately named the
bacteria the "Y2K bug."

All the while, Francis continued to follow Dr. Dixon's
work on the genetics of Treacher Collins syndrome. Since
his second year required that he give a graduate biology
seminar presentation to the entire department, this was the
topic he chose. Starting with the background of the syndrome, he went into great detail concerning its genetics
and its pathology. Of most interest to his audience was
his passion for the topic linked by his own personal life
experience. Both faculty and students engaged in asking
numerous questions at the end, which were recorded and
remain in his recording archives today.

In May 2001, Francis graduated for the second time
from IPFW, this time with a master's degree in biology.
Betty, Ruth, Susie, and her husband attended the ceremony,
followed by a small celebration, complete with a cake with
the black-and-yellow Purdue University crest on it.

Complete Surrender

Meanwhile, in graduate school, Francis set about applying again to medical schools. To help prepare for the retake of the MCAT, he heard about and signed up for a series of intensive weekly MCAT preparation classes that were held at the Indiana University Medical Center. With the guidance of his Indiana vocational rehab counselor, he was approved to have the course paid for along with reimbursement for his weekly drive and hotel stay in Indianapolis. From January through April, he made the two-and-a-half-hour trek with overnight stays in Indianapolis every weekend for the all-day Saturday classes. For eight hours, he sat through intensive review lectures on biology, chemistry, and physics and worked through countless practice problems in the science and math portions and wrote essays in the language and critical thinking portions. Practice mini-exams were given on a regular basis.

Francis took advantage of the AMCAS application to target a large number of schools across the United States. Once again, he was invited back to interview at IUSM, this time by two faculty doctors who took a genuine interest in his life experiences, goals, and interests along with his academic progress. When the doctors learned of his artistic side, he was asked to draw an anatomical sketch of a hand. The doctors were duly impressed.

After a long brutal wait filled with endless hope and ceaseless prayers, Francis received the letter he knew would make or break his dream of becoming a doctor. He was so apprehensive about the news that was inside the envelope he waited for Betty to come home so she could open it. As soon as she walked into the door, she could sense her son's great unease. Seeing the envelope on the table, her own heart was beating so hard her heart felt like it was going to jump out of her chest. Putting on her best smile, she calmly picked up the envelope and opened it. In seconds, her face crumpled. She didn't have to say a word as tears gathered at the corners of her eyes. Gathering her voice, she read the letter out loud where Francis learned that he was rejected by all the medical schools he had applied to. Devastated, he withdrew and sank inward while he processed the disappointment and reality that his years-long dream of becoming a doctor had come to an end.

***

Some time passed before Francis finally mustered up the courage to ask the Indiana University admissions tutor why. He was told that because of his hearing and speech disabilities, the corporate concern was he would not be able to communicate with his patients in the way.

Francis was not only crushed, he felt completely defeated and disoriented. If ever there was a time for soul-searching, it was now. After some serious time alone with the LORD, Francis prayerfully asked Him to unveil His will for his life. Even though his own heart's desire was in disarray, he fully trusted that the LORD's plan for his life were perfect. Even though he struggled mightily with the disappointing news, Francis willingly and completely surrendered himself to the LORD. It took some time, but finally, a sense of great peace came over him as he was led to apply to medical schools in Ireland and the United Kingdom that included applying for a biomedical science degree program from King's College in order to increase his chances.

Once again, Francis settled in for a long wait while his numerous applications were processed. All he could do was wait on the LORD and pray.

Chapter 4

The Longest Yard
2001

Heartbreak of a Nation

While driving from Garrett to Fort Wayne down State Road 327, Francis was enjoying an especially beautiful day. He was on his daily drive to work at the IPFW library, a job he had been holding down since 2000. On the car radio, he began hearing scattered sketchy reports of an airplane that crashed into one of the Twin Towers. At first, the report came in that it was a "small plane." Updated reports quickly followed. The plane was allegedly now an Airbus. Next, the second tower was hit, and the new report was both planes were "Boeing 767s from United and American Airlines." While he was listening, it was reported live that the first tower then the next collapsed. Like millions and millions of other Americans and billions of others around the world, he was shocked to his core and finding it difficult to grasp what was happening. His mind went immediately to the wonderful memory of the afternoon he spent at the World Trade Center. In that excruciating moment, he was so thankful that he had taken a few extra moments before he left the Observation Deck to turn around and take in and remember absolutely everything of that special visit as he could. Very clearly, he remembered the faces of those who sold him his souvenirs and the servers in the restaurant he ate at, all of those poor people who were all so kind and gracious to him. By now, he was in tears. He couldn't believe it!

Then more ominous reports began to flood in. The Pentagon was hit and was burning! Another report came that a flight had gone down in a field in rural Pennsylvania. America was under terrorist attack!

Somehow, Francis made it to campus. Somewhere along the way, he noticed the sky was completely clear of aircraft. Even the birds had stopped singing. When he arrived at the interlibrary loan office, the radio coverage continued. The FAA had grounded all aircraft under as a federal emergency order. A pair of F-16 fighters, likely armed, from the Fort Wayne airport's Air National Guard base circled like buzzards overhead. In downtown Fort Wayne, office towers were evacuated as a precaution.

Later on that day, there was a run on gas stations as prices skyrocketed to five dollars per gallon in some areas. When Francis returned home that evening, Betty was in a state of shock. As soon as he walked inside the door, she ran up to him and gave him a hug. She was so relieved he was home safe she wouldn't let go of him. For the rest of the day, they kept a vigil around the television for the ongoing coverage. Betty eventually sent him out that evening to get her yellow Beetle gassed up at the local Marathon where a line of cars curled out into the street while waiting for their turn at the pump. The tragedy of 9/11 was the equivalent of Pearl Harbor for Francis's generation.

A New Sideline

A lesson Americans always take to heart is that when tragedy strikes, you brush yourself off and pick yourself up and move forward as quickly as you can, and that's exactly what America—including Francis—did.

In the late summer of 2001, Francis considered taking up the acoustic guitar, so he went guitar shopping at several music shops in Fort Wayne. He settled on a beautiful new Epiphone Hummingbird guitar at a music store near Fort Wayne's biggest shopping mall. As soon as he bought it, he sought a guitar teacher. For a year, he studied with a teacher who was also the leader of a local blues band, but since all the guy knew was blues (and couldn't read music himself), he looked again for a new teacher. Finally, in 2002, Francis found a more qualified classical guitar instructor, Bob Ferguson, who also had his own program, *Guitar Showcase*, on Fort Wayne's local National Public Radio (NPR) station. With this new teacher, Francis built a solid foundation in music reading and classical guitar playing.

Now that Francis had a guitar, he began taking it on family camping trips, as Christopher used to do in years past, so the family could sing along again. He also sometimes played his guitar in church—particularly at Christmastime—when the congregation sang along as he played "Silent Night."

God—The Master Artist

While Francis was waiting to hear from the numerous medical schools he applied to, Betty encouraged him to explore the possibility of using his artistic skills in the service of medicine, perhaps as a medical illustrator.

For the third time, Francis was back at IPFW, this time in the art department, which classified him as a "permanent fixture" on campus. In the fall of 2002, he began a series of art classes spread among drawing, painting, graphic arts, and photography, all in the factorylike art building on campus.

The bulk of Francis's classes were in drawing. One memorable drawing class focused on the human figure, complete with nude, mostly female, models. Betty began to notice that one night when her son returned home from school, his face was beet red.

"He came home, and he was still blushing. I thought he had a fever. 'Are you all right, Francis? Let me feel your head. Do you have a fever?' 'No, Mom,' he said." It took some prying, but Francis finally explained to her that he had to draw a woman in the nude from a live model. 'They had a model, and she had no clothes on, Mom.' He was frantic about it. I was proud that something like that bothered my son. I said, 'I'm sorry, that's just part of life, I guess.'"

But the lesson in external human anatomy from the artistic point of view was well learned. Eventually, he overcame his embarrassment and came to see the created human body as a glorious work of art from the Master Artist Himself, God. What Francis couldn't see quite yet was that the LORD was preparing him all along for the future He had in place for him. Francis was being well prepared for future studies in human anatomy in another part of the world. In time, he took other drawing classes focusing on perspective still life and even self-portrait drawing, real or imagined. One such self-portrait depicted him as a surgeon in an operating room, holding an anesthesia mask toward the viewer, clearly drawn from the patient's point of view. Another self-portrait that he imagined was of him in a suit and hat, walking across Westminster Bridge in London with Big Ben in the background. Pushing his creative boundaries, he often used an abstract technique that utilized hundreds of tiny shapes and patterns to form his own face.

Francis's most memorable drawing, however, was that of the grand piano standing in the lobby of the IPFW student union building. For that, he used a combination of India ink painting and drawing. Eventually, this work of art won a prize in a local art show and became Betty's favorite piece of his artwork. Today, it is framed and hung with pride in Betty's home.

Next came lessons in oil painting where Francis learned to prepare the canvas, mix the colors into endless shades, and apply them with brushes of variety of shapes and sizes. From there came acrylic painting. After Ruth mentioned that his portrait of a man ascending a stairway to heaven where the light that emanated from a heavenly portal resembled the flames of hell in her eyes, Francis temporarily set aside his painting tools after he completed art classes for when the right time came for him to resume painting. In photography class, he felt secure enough to eventually submit his work to local art fairs where he won a few prizes.

However, as much as art was proving to be a wonderful diversion while he waited to be accepted at a major medical college, it certainly was not his true passion in terms of a profession. It was, however, something Francis considered to be a God-given talent like music had evidenced itself in his life.

The Longest Yard

Try as he might, Francis struggled with the angst that came with such a long wait. His heart was set on becoming a doctor. However, around every corner, there seemed to be another rejection and more disappointment waiting for him with very long lapses of time in between. Afraid to get his hopes up, only to face being let down again, he constantly came up with new ways to pass the time in an effort to buoy his sinking spirits. By this time, he was putting more effort into preparing himself for another letdown than he was in daring to keep on hoping and praying that his dreams would be fulfilled. Although he was still strong in his faith, every day that passed by without the letter of acceptance to medical school only served to prepare him for the fact that his dream would never happen. It was a terrible dilemma and a constant battle to lean on and trust in the LORD. In spite of it all and with the constant prayers of his mother and others, he hung on with all his might. So, during the interim, Francis planned a trip to Ireland.

Book 5

Trust in the Lord with all thine heart; and lean not unto thine own understanding and he shall direct thy paths.

—Proverbs 3:5–6 (King James Version)

Chapter 1

Ireland—Home Sweet Ancestral Home
2002

Once you're here, there's no goin' back.
—King Brian, King of the Leprechauns

Francis yearned to visit his ancestral home, Ireland. In 2002 when Francis set about applying to medical schools in Ireland and England, he also made plans to visit them.

Around his birthday in late April, he booked flights from Fort Wayne to Chicago to Dublin, Ireland, round-trip. His plan was to visit Trinity College Dublin, University College Dublin, and one other medical school in the city.

When Francis arrived at the Fort Wayne airport on the morning of his trip, he found the small airport terminal heavily guarded by the National Guardsmen with M-16 assault rifles stationed around the single security checkpoint, manned by the newly formed, federally run TSA, where he was thoroughly searched from top to bottom.

At Chicago O'Hare airport, Francis could not have been more excited when he was transferred to the new international terminal where he boarded the green Aer Lingus jet for Dublin. The in-flight movie was Disney's *Darby O'Gill and the Little People*. He fell asleep with a deep contented smile on his face.

Franny Boy

After a cheery immigration officer cleared him upon arrival in Dublin, he walked outside the terminal to catch his ride into Dublin.

As soon as Francis alighted from his transport in central Dublin, he stopped in his tracks. The sounds, the air, the smells, the people, and the architecture seemed eerily familiar to him. Almost immediately, he was hit by the strangest sensation; Ireland was home! The tune of "Danny Boy" swirled through his mind.

Oh, Franny Boy, the pipes, the pipes are calling
From glen to glen and down the mountainside.
The summer's gone, and all the roses are falling.
It's you, it's you, must go, and I must bide,
But come ye back when summer's in the meadow
Or when the valley's hushed and white with snow.
I'll be here in sunshine or in shadow.
Oh, Franny Boy, I love you so,
But if you come, and all the flowers are dying
And I am dead, as dead I well may be,

You'll come and find the place where I am lying
And kneel and say "Ave" there for me.
And I will rest in peace until you come to me.

Tears streamed down his face.

***

Regardless of the fact that he was completely exhausted, Francis went to the Sunday morning mass at the Christchurch Anglican cathedral in central Dublin. While standing for the entrance procession with the crucifix, he fell asleep, and he nearly toppled over into the aisle like a felled tree had it not been for a gracious churchgoer who caught him just in time. Realizing just how extremely tired he really was, he immediately went to the hotel, a beautiful independent hotel, where he checked in. His room was about the size of a small closet; it was barely large enough for a single bed with an en-suite bathroom.

Darby O'Gill and the Little People

At last, his head hit his pillow, and he faded into a deep dreamy sleep. He slumbered for hours before a wily old codger pulled off his covers and demanded that he get up. The gray-haired old man with thick gray bushy eyebrows and neatly trimmed moustache and beard looked vaguely familiar to him. Next to the old man was the tiniest little humanlike creature he had ever laid eyes on. He was only twenty-one inches tall! Who—what—on earth was he?

351

The old man bellowed in his thick Irish brogue, "Your lordship, why didn't ye tell us ye were comin'? I'd have opened the manor house for you."

Francis rubbed the sleep out of his eyes. His eyes darted back and forth between the old man and the little human creature. "Who are you?" he asked. "What are you doing here?"

"Darby O'Gill. We met on the flight. What ails you?" O'Gill leaned in as close to Francis as he could and whispered into his ear, "We've got to find a pot o' gold before"—he glanced at King Brian—"he does!"

Francis heard every word the old codger said, and he didn't even have his hearing aid on! He couldn't take his eyes off the tiny man with the big fat smirk on his face.

"You're looking at Brian of Knocknasheega, king of all the Leprechauns!"

King Brian stared straight back at Francis. "Three wishes I'll grant ye, great wishes an' small! But you wish a fourth, an' you'll lose them all!"

Darby O'Gill looked at Francis with mischief in his eyes. "Let me tell ye about me friend Billy. He asked me what was the quickest way into Cork. I said, 'Ye going by foot or by car?' Billy said, 'In the car.'"

"'Well,' I said, 'that's the quickest.'" Darby O'Gill and King Brian doubled over in laughter.

***

From his "home base," he spent the next three days visiting all three medical schools, most notably Trinity

College Dublin with its famous library housing the illuminated *Book of Kells* (sometimes referred to as the *Book of Columba* where the four gospels were contained in Latin), and visiting with some of the admissions tutors as the schools. He even braved visiting the anatomy dissection theatre at one of them. In between, he explored Dublin by bus and on foot where he walked along the River Liffey, through Temple Bar, and along Grafton Street, which was for pedestrians only. Unexpectedly, Francis was treated to an outstanding musical performance by a woman who had set up her grand piano on the street. Not surprisingly, he met many warm and friendly people. His new connection to his ancestral homeland was unbreakable.

Renewed Faith

Upon returning home, Francis was on a high he had never experienced before. For some strange reason, all felt right with his world, and even the thought of another possible disappointment couldn't shake it. In fact, he barely even thought about it.

That was a good thing. Shortly after his return home, Francis received the news that he was not accepted at any of the schools in Ireland he applied to. Albeit disappointed, he wasn't anywhere nearly as devastated as he was after learning he would never become a doctor. Instead, he welcomed the news with praise and gratitude for the visit to his ancestral homeland he had just been given. For him, visiting his ancestral homeland was the best birthday gift in his twenty-seven years he could ever have imagined, and regardless, his high could not be shaken. He picked himself up and brushed himself off, and with renewed faith, he aimed toward the door the LORD was about to open.

Chapter 2

The LORD Reveals His Will
2003

The letter from King's College London, the very last college he had applied to, arrived that afternoon, but Francis waited until he was in the kitchen with his mother before mentioning it. He placed it on the counter then said to Betty, "Aren't you going to open it?"

Francis appeared nonchalant, but Betty knew he was putting on an act. This was it. Trying to squelch her own queasiness, she opened the letter and read it to herself. Her eyes went wide, and her face was consumed by a huge grin. Then she squealed! King College London was offering him a place in the biomedical sciences degree program! Although this was not medical school, per se, it was a great opportunity for a career in medical research. The LORD's plan was unfolding! After years and months of clinging to hope, in that moment, Francis experienced an indescribable perfect peace about his future. After giving thanks and praise to the LORD, he wasted no time accepting the offer that was, in British parlance, an unconditional offer, based on his past academic performance. On the form, there was an option to accept his place for entry that year, 2003, or to defer entry for the following year. The British call this one-year deferral the "gap year." Francis chose to defer because he knew he needed the time to prepare for his first move away from home, clear across the Atlantic Ocean. In order to prepare for his college time in London, Francis planned a springtime visit to London, where he would be residing for three years. Included in his agenda was a side trip to Manchester to visit Dr. Dixon at the University of Manchester where he had his own laboratory.

Across the River Thames

Once Francis was accepted at King's College London, he made arrangements with the King's admissions tutor, Dr. Kevin O'Byrne, for a tour of the campus. King's College, begun in 1829, was now a part of the University of London and has multiple campuses scattered throughout central London. The campus he visited would be the one he would be attending the following year—Guy's Hospital—that is located on the south bank of the River Thames, near the Tower Bridge and across the river from the Tower of London. The Guy's campus is a sprawling collection of imposing buildings, the oldest dating from 1721, when the hospital was founded. There are other buildings on the campus, some dated from the nineteenth century and newer ones built in the late twentieth century.

One building, a solid concrete tower called Guy's Tower, is the world's tallest hospital at thirty-four stories. Built in 1975, an opinion that is shared by many architectural critics, it is a perfect example of Soviet-style brutalist architecture. Some locals refer to it as London's ugliest building.

The newest building on campus, New Hunt's House, was built in the late nineties and was where Francis would attend lectures and laboratory training. New Hunt's House sported an interesting architectural feature: on a set of tall vertical glass panels in front of the west entrance, DNA double helix and other images from the world of biomedical sciences were etched into the glass.

Francis's deep love for architecture was certainly being satisfied at King's College, an added bonus he hadn't given any conscious thought of. The day spent with Dr. O'Byrne had given him far more than he expected, and he was more convinced than ever this is where the LORD intended for him to be.

For the rest of the week, Francis visited all the popular tourist attractions, but what excited him the most were the several medical museums he somehow managed to find. Across the street from Guy's Hospital campus was the old St. Thomas Church, built in the early nineteenth century. Upstairs, at the end of a creaky old wooden spiral staircase going up the steeple to the attic, was a little museum containing a medicinal herb garret, medical history displays, and the main attraction, the restored 1822 operating amphitheater with a steep roof skylight. Evidently, this was part of the original St. Thomas Hospital that had been combined with the original Guy's Hospital. The women's operating theatre was located in the attic of the church and was originally connected to the old St. Thomas Hospital, which was, by now, long gone. Wooden stands arranged in a horseshoe allowed doctors and students to watch the operation in progress. In the center was a crude wooden operating table that was surrounded by some chairs. By its side was a cabinet for surgical instruments. If you stand in the theatre, completely silent, you can hear the screams of agony while some poor pregnant woman endured a cesarean section without any anesthesia. Surgeries were brutal and agonizing in those days. Amputations, he was told, were done in record time in order to minimize the shock and pain as much as humanly possible. Francis couldn't help but shudder just thinking about it! The next hospital museum he visited, St. Bartholomew's Hospital, was far tamer, for which he was thankful. The dungeons of the Tower of London paled by comparison, Francis thought.

Thankfully, the Crown Jewels and throne rooms were a welcome reprieve from the brutality of archaic preanesthetic surgeries. Francis did give it some serious thought that modern-day medicine was a cakewalk compared to two centuries ago. He promised himself no matter what he needed to endure in the way of more surgeries, he would never ever complain after seeing what some people, who had no choice, had to suffer through.

***

The guided tour of the Tower with the Beefeaters was a welcome relief. The tour of the Tower was not complete until he visited the Tower Bridge and watched the drawbridge open up and saw the engine room that controlled the drawbridge. He enjoyed the Tate Modern art gallery. But the most impressive part of his London week was attending the Sunday evening Eucharist in Westminster Abbey. Francis was completely blown away by its majesty, and he couldn't shake the sensation that he was in God's throne room itself. However, his trip would not be considered to be officially over until he visited the Old Curiosity Shop in London, not only for its literary importance but also because his father had once bought some miniature etchings and plaques from there during his service in World War II. Built in Shakespeare's time and immortalized by Charles Dickens, it was sadly now a shoe repair shop.

A Side Trip to Manchester

Saving the most anticipated part of his trip for last, Francis said goodbye to London and caught a train bound for Manchester for a visit to Dr. Dixon and his wife Jill. The Dixons were a research team, and they showed him around their lab at the University of Manchester where he was introduced to the students and postdocs who worked there. The Dixons talked at great length about their work on the gene for Treacher Collins syndrome genetics. Only then was his trip officially over. From Manchester, he flew to Chicago, then onto Fort Wayne. The trip had laid a firm foundation for his future.

Wrapping Up the Gap Year

In the fall of 2003, Francis gratefully endured another surgery. The implantable hearing aid he wore dated back to 1987, and it was now on its last legs. Dr. Tubergen, who had tried to surgically open his ear canals in 1978 but could not because of the severity of the deformity of his middle ear cavities, now had a private practice in Indianapolis. Francis was hopeful that, because surgical techniques had advanced sufficiently since then, there was a real possibility that could happen. However, Dr. Tubergen nixed the idea of another surgical attempt to open his ear canal for the same previous reasons, but he did recommend a new more advanced type of hearing aid called the bone-anchored hearing aid or "BAHA." This is a two-part hearing device. One part is a tiny screw that is drilled through the skin into the mastoid bone behind the ear. The other piece is a small sound processor that snaps onto the external part of the screw. There would no longer be a need for a bulky body-worn battery pack and cords, which was quite obtrusive. The small sound processor of the new hearing aid picks up sound and transmits it directly into the bone through the screw, which sets up vibration and resonance in the skull, much like the body of a guitar or violin resonates when the strings are played. Immediately, he decided to go ahead with Dr. Tubergen's recommendation and scheduled the surgery for late September 2003.

Comparatively speaking, this surgery was easier on Francis than many of his others had been. (After all, he had just witnessed what ancient, archaic surgeries used to be like, and no way was he about to complain!) Quickly, he was rendered unconscious via Propofol that was injected into his IV. The anesthesiologist inserted a new type of breathing tube with a pig-snout end that went over the opening to his trachea and could be blindly inserted. Suddenly, he was out like a light. With that accomplished, Dr. Tubergen made a tiny hole in his right temple and drilled into the bone. He drove the tiny screw into the bone then put the external piece on it with the skin around it. Francis awakened not too long after this short procedure, and he was released to go home where he slept soundly for the rest of the day and all through the night.

A month later, the bone had healed securely enough around the screw to allow for the new BAHA "box" behind the ear. Once it was snapped into place on the screw and turned on, there was a whole world of difference between his old clunker hearing aids and his new one. Not to mention, it didn't scream "handicapped" when one happened to see it. The old clunkers, of course, ended up in his personal medical archives collection.

The rest of the gap year served Francis well as he was able to devote the entire year for getting the necessities done for his upcoming future in London. First on the agenda was to secure the necessary funding via student loans for a minimum of three years for both tuition and living expenses. Letters were needed explaining what funding would support him for the duration of the course in order to satisfy the United Kingdom immigration officials. Also needed was to renew his passport and get his U.K. international student visa, also known as the U.K. Entry Clearance for Students, which was good for three years. As soon as he received his new passport, he sent it to the British consulate via FedEx to get the U.K. student visa.

The summer of 2004 was one of Francis's busiest and most bittersweet ever. After all, in order to move forward into his new life adventure, he was also preparing to depart from friends and family he had known since the beginning of his life with the Smiths. Betty had broken her foot, so he and Ruth doted on her while she healed. (Looking back, Betty believes that God was telling her to slow down.) For whatever reason, Ruth and Francis decided the house needed some updating. Some of the rooms were repainted, and in others, along with a friend, they tore up all the carpeting in the front foyer, parlor, and side room and sanded and finished the pine floor in the parlor and the rooms on either side of the parlor. Pergo laminate flooring was then laid in the foyer and in one of the side rooms. That September, many of their lifelong friends gathered to celebrate Betty's eightieth birthday at the Red Cedar horse farm and therapeutic riding facility outside Fort Wayne with lots of food and fellowship. That fall, Francis gave his final notice at his IPFW library job, and his co-workers threw him a bon voyage farewell party in celebration of his new journey and new life overseas. As his last Sunday drew near, he bade farewell to everyone at Lakewood Park Baptist Church.

A Frightening Malady

There was still one medical issue that was growing in seriousness that Francis had to tackle before he left for England. Because of his lower jaw deformity and upper airway obstruction, he was unable to breathe properly at night, hence his terrible rattling snoring. Over the past few years, his condition worsened to the point he could not stay awake during the day. He would fall asleep during the day anytime, anywhere while driving or in church or class. Between wakefulness and full sleep, bizarre twilight dreams permeated his semiconscious state. Gasping for breath is what usually awakened him, accompanied by killer headaches that made him dry heave or heave up acid in the middle of the night or early morning. Numerous physicians were consulted, but none of them was able to do much more than prescribe medications from Ritalin to Provigil, both stimulants, to help him stay awake during the day. Nothing worked. His immediate concern was that he was not getting enough oxygen at night, which he mentioned to his doctors. Finally, the LORD led him to a doctor who was able to shed some light on his mystery problem. He was given a pulse oximeter that is used to measure oxygen levels in the blood to wear while he was sleeping. The low blood oxygen saturation level was so alarming he was immediately referred to a pulmonary and critical care specialist who met with him right away. The specialist, who was in Fort Wayne, wasted no time in sending him to Parkview Hospital for an overnight sleep study.

Francis went to sleep that night in the hospital's sleep lab, trussed up like a turkey with wires all over his head that were connected to a machine. The findings were alarming. He stopped breathing upward of two hundred times that night, and the seriously life-threatening low oxygen in his blood was finally confirmed. Not wasting any time, he was instructed to come back to the hospital that night for another sleep test with a breathing machine. The next day, the pulmonologist diagnosed him with severe obstructive sleep apnea where his upper airway was blocked by the tongue or other tissue while he slept. This was a potentially fatal disease if not caught in time. Betty recalled the time when she and Francis visited Ruth at her university and they were sleeping overnight in her apartment. She became alarmed when he woke her up, fighting and convulsing in his sleep because he wasn't getting enough air. Immediately after his sleep studies, Francis was prescribed a special breathing machine called a continuous positive airway pressure (CPAP) machine, a type of respirator that forces air at high pressure into the airway to keep it from collapsing as his always did. After the machine was calibrated and fitted to him, he slept for what seemed like years for the first time in his life. Since the machine breathed for him, he now had a new lease on life. There is no doubt that, if the problem had not been caught by that time, he surely would have died in his sleep before too long. Once again, the LORD intervened.

Betty Cries Buckets

Secure in knowing that a major health crisis was averted, Francis faced his immediate future with great excitement and joy. He was *free*!

For the rest of his short time at home, Francis began the tedious task of packing two large suitcases with the clothes he would need in London along with other items he needed. The CPAP had dual voltage so he could travel anywhere with it. Shortly before he left for London, he, Betty, and Ruth spent one last weekend at Purdue University with Ruth where they attended a home football game. Ruth gave him a Curious George in a space suit to take with him. Curious George received "first class" travel seating in one of the open side pockets of his rollaboard backpack (as a carry-on bag) where he would travel alongside his master while flying over the pond.

Francis's last night at home in Garrett was a bittersweet one. His friend John Sargent, with whom he did his music ministry at the county farm on Sundays after church, came over with his wife, as did Becky and her husband. Betty, as usual, cooked one of her magnificent meals. Through happy tears, hugs, and farewells, he was bid bon voyage. No one knew really when he would be back home again. After packing up last-minute items, such as his piano music, he went to bed early, as did Betty and Ruth. They had to arise at three thirty in the morning for the six-o'clock-in-the-morning flight to Chicago where he would connect to Pittsburgh for his overseas flight.

As "prepared" as they were, it was very difficult for all of them to leave the house for what was to be Francis's last time home for an indefinite time. Although he was outwardly excited, inwardly he was scared and uncertain. For all intents and purposes, he knew no one in London, so this definitely was a leap of faith. At this point, he could only trust in his LORD that this was His will for his life. Betty was completely torn up, and even though she tried to hide her feelings, she didn't do a very good job of it. With three bulging pieces of luggage crammed into his green Pontiac Bonneville along with Betty and Ruth, Francis drove through his neighborhood that was as dead and silent as a tomb. No one else was awake at that hour.

Even the airport was sleepy. After checking his bags, it felt like the walk to the security checkpoint was like walking his last mile. Since Betty and Ruth could not accompany Francis through security, they at least were able to stand in the security line with him. Finally, they had no other choice than to bid him farewell at the entrance, all of them doing little to choke back their tears. Betty told him, rather loudly, to behave himself around the cadavers. On the other side of the checkpoint, Francis turned and waved before walking off, in tears, to the gate. Before long, he was in the air, looking down at the Fort Wayne skyline, just as the sun was beginning to rise. Francis and Curious George were on their way!

Betty remembered, "I was so proud of him, but it was so hard to let him go." Francis later learned that when Betty got home, she had had a good cry and was practically inconsolable.

During the flight, Francis experienced the peace that came with knowing that at last he was in God's perfect will for his life. He had plenty of time to give gratitude and thanks for all the difficult trials the LORD had carried him through during his lifetime and for the numerous times the LORD said no to his desires because He knew all along that His plans were perfect. In hindsight, he could clearly see that the LORD was teaching him patience and to never give up on his goals. Now that he was on his way to his new life overseas, he was going to trust and depend on Him even more as He guided Francis through this yet-unknown territory. He had no idea what lay ahead of him, but the LORD did, and that was what mattered. There was no doubt in his mind that the LORD was taking him on the journey of a lifetime.

Book 6

Have I not commanded you? Do not be frightened, do not be dismayed, for the Lord your God is with you wherever you go.

—Joshua 1:9

Chapter 1

The Journey of a Lifetime
2004

The Great Cheery London Adventure—
and Music Galore

At the crack of dawn on a typical London foggy morning, Francis groggily awoke shortly before the plane landed at London's Gatwick Airport. Thankfully, he had actually been able to sleep on the plane. After collecting his humongous bags from baggage claim, he had to struggle to schlep all his stuff through Her Majesty's Customs and Immigration. When the cheery and very friendly immigration officer saw his U.K. entry clearance student visa that was good for three years, she asked him where he was going to go to school in London. When he answered, "King's College London," she smiled and wished him luck and told him she hoped he enjoyed his time in London as she stamped his passport. He took the Gatwick Express train from the airport to London's Victoria Station. Upon arrival there, he queued in line for one of the ubiquitous black taxis outside the station.

Boy, the people in London certainly were cheery! The older cheery gentleman cabbie chatted him up one side and down the other, asking him what he was going to do in London with all those bags! So far, Francis was batting a thousand with "cheery" Londoners!

At last, the taxi pulled up in front of Francis's new home—a large sprawling University of London residence hall named International Hall. Located in the Bloomsbury district, it was built in the early sixties for university students coming in from all over the world. The building was a mix of sixties and Georgian architecture and also had a new addition that was opened in 2003 by Her Majesty Queen Elizabeth II. This particular Hall of Residence served foreign students from all the colleges of the University of London, including King's. Once Francis had accepted King's offer for a residence, he received information on numerous halls. There were so many to choose from! He settled on International Hall not only because it was conveniently located in central London but also because it was catered, meaning it had a dining room and all meals were a part of his room and board fees. Besides the dining room, the hall also provided laundry facilities, music practice rooms with pianos, and a bar and lounge with an antique Broadwood grand piano, and two TV/cinema rooms.

In place of the larger two-to-four student dorm rooms found in U.S. university halls, this hall housed tiny single-person rooms referred to as "single study bedrooms."

Larger apartment-style accommodations were for married students. This was typical of British university halls, and this suited Francis just fine as he was accustomed to having his own room, like he did at home. After he checked in, he got settled into his "monk's cell" room on the second floor. The room had everything he needed—a twin bed, wardrobe, desk and chair with shelves above it, and a washbasin. A single window provided a nice light and a "view" of a Georgian brick building across the street. The toilet and shower were shared facilities located just a short distance down the hall. All in all, he was happily cozy. After all, this was going to be his home for the next three years.

The next morning, Monday, was a day that was fully devoted to registering as a new student at King's College London. First thing that morning, Francis arrived at Guy's Hospital campus for orientation lectures and introductions to his professors as well as the chaplaincy staff comprised of one Anglican chaplain and the other, a Catholic. Both would become close friends of Francis. After all the introductory formalities, he was processed through a series of registration steps, each one taking place in a separate room in order of the steps of registration. Eventually, he was provided with a photo ID, then proceeded to register for his first year "fresher" series of classes and tutorials, made up of small group mini-classes. At the financial office, he was asked to provide his student loan documentation. When it came time to purchase his numerous textbooks, the bookstore in the oldest part of the hospital's building was handy for him as most of his lectures for the first year were to be in physiology, pharmacology, histology, and other medical subjects, located in the main lecture theatre in the newest building, as were his laboratory sessions. Other lectures were held in the much older parts of the hospital that lent a historical charm to his experience.

The Cheery Little Maestro Strikes London

Now that the particulars were over and true to Francis's form, he didn't waste any time making new friends, most of whom were among his fellow students who resided in the hall. Being an "international" residence, his new friends were from all over the world: New Zealand, Taiwan, Greece, and guys from the Middle East and Europe. His best friend was a Greek woman named Mary, and the two became steadfast friends over the next three years. For hours at a time, he practiced on the upright pianos in the piano practice rooms. But his favorite was the antique Broadwood grand piano in the bar. He often entertained the bar crowd on it. This, he decided, was how he could keep up his piano-playing skills that otherwise would have rusted away.

Settling In

Another to-do list necessity was to find the proper and necessary medical care for himself. Since Francis would be living in the U.K. beyond the minimum six months required for health coverage, he was eligible for the National Health Service (NHS) socialized health care system. The university had a general practitioner's surgery (British speak for doctor's office) located on the main campus of King's College, on the Strand. Thus, his health issues were taken care of. The practitioner was duly worried though with his inability to keep a healthy weight on. The remedy? He was prescribed Ensure, British style. Unlike the U.S. where Ensure can be bought over the counter nicely packed in plastic containers, the U.K. Ensure was prescription only in old-style tin cans. Every month, he would have to carry a big box of it from Boots "chemist" (drugstore) shop to the hall.

What Francis missed terribly though was Betty's home cooking. Before too long, he discovered he was not quite enamored with the institutional food, and rather too quickly, he began to lose weight on what already was a seriously thin frame.

Thankfully, it turned out that he enjoyed British and Irish food, and both remain among his favorite cuisines today. There was also another obstacle he had to overcome; since the cafeteria food was rationed out to hundreds of students processing along the line, he had to rejoin the queue for seconds just to stay properly fed. Adding to this dilemma was the fact that he was an "eating machine." It took vast quantities of food to feed his overhyped metabolism. At times, it took him over two hours just to eat one meal. After a noticeable significant weight loss, some of the employees who came to know him well encouraged him to reenter the line just before last service in order to get seconds. Gradually, the lost weight came back on.

Wisely, Francis had the foresight to arrive in London a week before classes began. The next unanticipated challenge was to locate a special alarm clock for deaf people, one that had a loud, piercing alarm and had a vibrator device that was placed under the pillow. You would *think* that he would somehow be able to find one in a high-street (major shopping street) department store or electrical goods store, but that was not the case. After days of frustration and practically at zero hour, he located one through a British deaf council that sold them through their website.

The rest of Francis's first week was spent familiarizing himself with his surrounding neighborhoods. He thoroughly enjoyed himself walking around and taking the tube, trying to find his way from his hall in Bloomsbury to the Guy's Hospital campus of King's at London Bridge. Just across the street from the south side of his hall was London's original big children's hospital, Great Ormond Street Hospital for Children, founded in 1852.

***

It is difficult to surmise what Francis enjoyed the most—studying medical biology in the United Kingdom, its beautiful ancient architecture, or his ongoing love affair with music that he was developing to its fullest, not to mention his new eclectic group of outstanding friendships. Or perhaps it was his English breakfast that was composed of a wide slab of bacon, eggs, black pudding, toast and butter, and potatoes from his hall's cafeteria. Each day after breakfast, he rode the tube from Russell Square station, changed trains at King's Cross—St. Pancras station—and got off at London Bridge to walk across the skybridge connecting the railway station to the Guy's Hospital campus. Whatever his uncertainties were, they were shoved to the background without so much as a second thought as he quickly became acclimated to his new lifestyle and new friends.

Within weeks, Francis found himself playing the piano for Thursday evening Anglican service at Guy's Hospital chapel as a regular. He joined the Guys, King's, and St. Thomas's (GKT) Music Society—an orchestra composed of students, staff, and others from Guy's Hospital, King's College, and the St. Thomas Hospital medical and dental schools—as a pianist. For the Christmas concert, the group played at the nearby Southwark Cathedral, whose ancient cavernous Gothic structure provided the most wonderful resounding acoustics he had ever heard. Another concert was performed in 2005 at St. John's church near Waterloo Station, where Francis performed two piano solos.

Her Majesty Is Just Like Mom!

Another GKT society—the Surgical Society—provided the best training in surgical technique (incisions and suturing) as well as weekly lectures on surgical and related historical topics. Of course, Francis joined! Having become fast friends with both the Anglican and Catholic chaplains, he became involved with the chaplaincy of all the King's College London campuses. Each October, the chaplaincy held a religious and social retreat at Cumberland Lodge, a former royal residence that was built in 1650, that was turned into a conference lodge/hotel for university educational retreats on religious and societal issues after World War II, which Francis was very caught up in. Located in Windsor Park, the huge city-sized royal park that is home to Windsor Castle, this lodge boasted huge conference rooms, dining space, and gathering rooms complete with antique grand pianos, a soaring grand oak staircase, as well as several en-suite guest rooms. Its sheer size, as well as its expanse of meadows and woods, provided for splendid mosquitoless hikes. While there, he attended the Royal Chapel, a tiny stone church in one of the wooded areas that, on occasion, Her Majesty Queen Elizabeth II and other royals were known to attend.

During his next retreat to Cumberland Lodge one year later, Francis actually did catch a glimpse of Her Majesty Queen Elizabeth II and her consort Prince Phillip as they were getting into their Jaguar station wagon. As fate would have it, he actually got to meet them both! Again, it was at the retreat. After Francis and his group left the Royal Chapel, the royal couple emerged shortly after them. To this day, he has no idea what went on behind the scenes, but before he realized what was about to happen, his group was allowed to meet Her Majesty and Prince Phillip. One by one, their names were called. When it came time for his turn, he said his name then bowed, first to Her Majesty and then to Prince Phillip. The queen was as gracious as she was gorgeous, and all he could think of was how much

Her Majesty reminded him of his mother! Francis couldn't wait to call Betty to tell her just how much he thought Queen Elizabeth reminded him of her. Betty was terribly flattered and still laughs about that phone call to this day. For Francis, the memory of that remarkable experience is as clear and vivid to him as the day it happened. Looking back, he can only chalk this experience up as fate.

Joyous Excursions

Even on weekends, Francis kept himself busy. The time was used to explore London in greater depth, usually off the beaten path. Over time, he explored the Science Museum plus others, including Greenwich's Maritime Museum, the clipper sailing ship *Cutty Sark*, the London Transport Museum, and too many others to list. Adding to his delight, he discovered that London itself was home to numerous other small museums relating to medicine, surgery, anesthesia, and anatomy. Never before had he observed another city on earth that was devoted to such a preponderance of museums devoted strictly to medicine! He even revisited the Old Operating Theatre, the restored 1820s operating amphitheater in the attic of St. Thomas Church. The list of medical museums was endless, each one more fascinating than the others. Oh, one can only imagine being a terrified patient about to undergo such torturous, painful procedures.

Along the way, Francis discovered great joy in other excursions, most notably antiquing. He loved to stroll through the antique markets that sprang up along both sides of Portobello Road on Saturdays. He got to know several of the vendors well, including those who sold him his prized pieces for his medical collection that included a nineteenth-century tracheostomy surgical set in a black box, a tonsillotome that was basically a guillotine for tonsillectomy, and other antique surgical instruments.

Plane spotting was always one of Francis's favorite pastimes back home in Indiana, and his passion for it revived itself in London in no time at all on clear sunny days. Heathrow Airport was just an hour's ride on the Picadilly line of the tube from the hall, so, along with several other men, they gathered at a particular spot around the airport perimeter, off the runway end, to spot incoming or outgoing aircraft. While many, including Francis, pointed their cameras upward, others had little notebooks where tail numbers and models of aircraft were recorded while they swept skyward and came down from the sky to land. It was a fascinating "hobby" of sorts and certainly one he never grew tired of. Years later as he was perusing his memorabilia of his time in the U.K., he came across boxes upon boxes of images of Boeing 747s, 777s, and other wide-body jets, as well as rare visitors such as government VIP aircraft and private 747s from the Middle East, experimental aircraft, new models, and rugged-looking Soviet-built airliners. The list was endless, each of them equally fascinating. Regrettably, he missed out on seeing the supersonic Concorde in flight, but time permitting, he would visit vintage airports complete with preserved aircraft. While in London, whenever he heard the whine of a jet engine overhead, he couldn't help but stop, look up, and identify the aircraft that was overhead. There was no end to his aircraft curiosity.

A Christmas Carol

Before Francis knew it, it was Christmastime in 2004. Knowing that he could not possibly make it home was a huge disappointment for him. Thankfully, through the Host U.K. program that was designed to match international students in U.K. universities with host families, he was eventually matched with an older couple living in the small town of Camborne, in Cornwall. Two days before Christmas, he took a five-hour train ride from London's Paddington station across the southern England countryside to Cornwall, located in the extreme southwest point of England surrounded by the Atlantic. His older host couple was Mr. and Mrs. Cocup, who picked him up at Camborne's station where they subsequently drove him to their bungalow at the edge of town. In short order, Francis learned they were both taking lessons in brass instruments, and they had an upright piano in their home.

After getting Francis settled, Mr. and Mrs. Cocup then drove him around the area, stopping to visit the seaside towns of Mousehole and Penzance. While walking along the sea-battered cliffs along the Atlantic Ocean, he noticed a lighthouse out on its own island in the ocean, standing up to the battering of waves, its beams of light piercing holes in the cloud cover. An unexpected strong gust of wind would have blown him over had it not been for his hosts grabbing and hanging onto him for dear life. Later on, he could only imagine them trying to explain to Betty how the winds carried her son away.

Christmas traditions in the U.K. are unlike those practiced in the U.S. Although steeped into the heart of Francis that Christmas was a joyous day of celebrating the birth of Jesus, his LORD and Savior, he thoroughly embraced the traditions of his host country, which were slightly more formal and not as crass and commercial as it sometimes could be back home. There were similarities though.

Traditionally, Christmas Eve is a day of family, baking cookies, wrapping gifts, and hanging stockings over the fireplace that blazes with the Yule log. Then the family gathers around the Christmas tree while someone narrates their favorite story of all, Charles Dickens's *A Christmas Carol.*

Since the Cocups' children would not arrive until Christmas Day, the threesome enjoyed their own day of Christmas music of their own making before attending the midnight Eucharist at Camborne's Anglican parish church, St. Martin and St. Meriadoc. Nothing was more beautiful to Francis than hearing the wonderful Christmas carols that heralded the birth of Christ sung in the church by the choir and congregation, accompanied by a massive pipe organ. He truly felt the presence of Jesus stirring deep into his soul.

On Christmas Day, the couple's children and relatives arrived for dinner, which was a lovely fare of baked ham and mulled wine with small traditional homemade pies filled with nuts and dried fruits. The day was massive fun celebrating Christmas and watching the excited children emptying their Christmas stockings and unwrapping their presents under the tree. Christmas truly was a joyous occasion for Francis and the Cocup family.

Missing his mother and Ruth, Francis called home, allowing Betty to hear from her son and for Ruth to hear from her brother from overseas, which was both a joyous and bittersweet call. Both Betty and Ruth missed him as much as he missed them, terribly! Christmas at home simply was not the same without Francis. The day after Christmas in the U.K. is Boxing Day, a national holiday. With great reluctance, he bade farewell to his gracious hosts and headed back to London where he resumed swotting (studying) for the semester's final exams after the holidays.

"Whenever Francis is in London, he looks up the Cocups," mentioned Betty. Betty feels enormously blessed by the so many wonderful people who loved and looked after her son and that Francis was able to find such a lovely, caring family to spend Christmas with. He remains close to the Cocups to this day.

When Francis returned to his dormitory room and settled in, he couldn't help but reflect on how blessed he was to have spent his first Christmas overseas and away from his family with as warm and as special a family as the Cocups. Reflecting on his journey to where he was in that moment, he could clearly see that no time was ever wasted during the years of his journey. Instead, through trials and disappointments, prayer and faith, each and every step of the way was ordained by the LORD for the very special plans He had all along for Francis.

Chapter 2

Back to Work

Semester Finals

The New Year of 2005 was ushered in by a blazing display of fireworks exploding over the Houses of Parliament as Big Ben struck midnight. Among the crowd (akin to New York's Times Square) that gathered along the northern bank of the Thames, Francis watched the unfolding display with great awe. On New Year's Day, he joined the throngs of people that gathered in Trafalgar Square as a parade (which included a high school marching band from Indiana) marched by.

Christmas break came to an end, and with it came the arduous task of study time for the first semester's finals for all of Francis's classes. These exams were off campus, and for a week, give or take, he traveled across London to the Victoria Embankment area where there were two large gymnasium-sized exhibition halls called the Royal Horticultural Halls, where all the university final exams were traditionally administered. Their cavernous interiors were filled with ranks and files of desks with a dais at the front of the room on which sat the main invigilator (proctor) of the examination. Starting time was announced, and students busied themselves with exam papers and the blue essay books put before them. A handful of the invigilator's assistants strolled between the columns of desks. Exam times have a bad habit of seeming too short, and all too soon, time would be called, and their papers and blue essay books were surrendered to the invigilators as the students filed out.

The next semester began shortly after the exams, and that's when the students received their marks. To his enormous relief, Francis learned he had done quite well. For the rest of the next semester, students continued on with the same courses since they were term courses and not just for the semester.

The Green Violin

Sometime during the previous months, Francis discovered a unique music store named Hobgoblin Music, on Rathbone Place, a side street off Oxford Street. This unique shop specialized in traditional ethnic folk instruments from around the world. On the wall was a vast array of violins that were varnished in a rainbow of translucent colors. Next to a black violin were a purple, blue, red, pink, and even a green violin. Over the years while he still lived in Indiana, he had attempted to play the violin, but over and over, he failed to get any sound out of it. (It turns out the rosin that came with the violins was too hard and dry to use on the bow for friction.) However, after a few months of regular visits to this unusual shop, Francis gave into temptation, and he bought the green violin along with

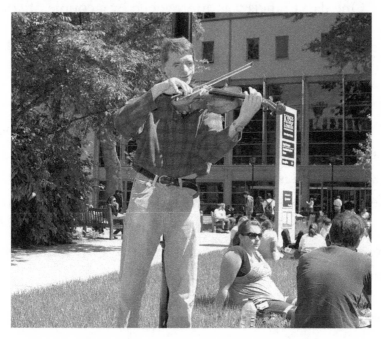

The Green Violin concert along the River Thames.
Francis acquired many devoted fans.

a how-to booklet that explained the mechanics and fundamentals of the instrument. From that point on, he was on his way. The fingering wasn't at all difficult since it was fairly similar to that of guitar playing, but the bowing and tone production were slightly more of a challenge. To teach himself the music, he took some existing piano music and rewrote it for violin. So enthralled was he with his musical new accomplishment that he parked himself on the South Bank of the Thames, near the Shakespeare's Globe Theatre, where he began to play. Soon, he was a regular, and he gathered quite an adoring crowd and soon who delighted in listening to his music.

One day, Francis was approached by a couple of tourists. One of them asked him what was the quickest way to Buckingham Palace.

"Ye going by foot or by car?" asked Francis.

"In the car," replied the tourist.

"Well," answered Francis, "that's the quickest!" Francis doubled over in laughter. Francis's street display of his green violin music paid off. In one day, he actually earned twenty-five pounds, about forty-five U.S. dollars. To this day, the Green Violin is synonymous with Francis as he rarely goes anywhere without it and plays it wherever and whenever he can.

Finding Bob's World War II History

One adventure Francis longed for was to locate his father's former World War II U.S. Army Air Base. That spring, along with the help of the Royal Air Force Museum historians, Bob's Eighth Air Force's 490th Bomb Group Base was located near the village of Eye, in the country of Suffolk in the northeast section of England. The nearest city was Norwich.

One Friday after spring final exams, Francis boarded a train from London to Norwich where he found himself a hotel for a weekend visit in order to find the base. The RAF museum staff went one step further; they referred him to a sweet elderly couple that had lived in the area their entire lives. They met Francis at the train station and drove him around the Suffolk countryside and on to Eye, where they visited the town parish church. There, in the church, was a memorial to the 490th Bomb Group's men! Francis found his father's name there along with quite a few photos of all the men. This was an emotional moment for him to see his father's honor memorialized in such a public and meaningful way. From there, the couple drove him to the remains of the airbase itself. The main runway was still there, and some weed-overgrown remote concrete hardstands and rusty Quonset huts were all that was left from the war. Flanking the runway were several newer warehouses. He stood on the runway and took some photos. Close by the base was a pub whose proprietors remembered the men who frequented it during the war. Although Bob was not specifically remembered, there was little doubt in Francis's mind that his father very well could have joined his buddies there after their missions. On a personal level, the visit to his father's old wartime base was his most memorable of all his experiences during the three years He spent in the U.K.

Home for the Summer and God's Divine Intervention

No one was more excited for summer to arrive than Betty. For the first time since Francis left for the U.K., he was coming home for summer. That June, after his spring exams, he traveled home to a very joyous reunion. While on the plane heading westbound, he couldn't help but bow his head to give thanks to his LORD for all that He had made possible for him and for his safety during his journey.

Little did Francis know that, by coming home when he did, he avoided a tragedy, one that very likely would have killed him. On July 7, 2005, an Islamic terror group struck London. The London Tube was bombed as well as some of the public transport buses. Fifty-six innocent lives were taken on the Piccadilly line, the very one Francis took to classes every day. Ruth was the first one to hear about it on the radio, information she quickly passed on to her brother. As soon as Betty was informed of the attack, she collapsed in a chair and gave thanks to the LORD for protecting her son. Betty prayed diligently and ceaselessly for her son's safety and protection while he was away from home, and in that moment, she knew the LORD answered her prayers. Right then and there, Betty made him promise that he would never go in the tube again. Betty said, "I knew when he promised me he wouldn't, he would keep his promise." Thankfully, it being summertime, no one he knew was involved in the bombing, and for that, he was extremely grateful. Still, he couldn't help but feel sad and heartbroken over the loss of so many innocent lives. More than ever before, Francis was reminded that when he was walking with the LORD and ensconced in the LORD's plan for his life, God's hand was constantly protecting him.

***

Other than that terrific upset, Francis enjoyed his quiet summer break. It was a time of catching up on family and friends and church family in the Fort Wayne area. Betty, Ruth, and Francis took a camping trip to Chain O'Lakes with the older but smaller Dodge motor home Betty had purchased two years prior. It was great for camping, especially as it had electrical outlets for Francis's CPAP. Together, they visited their old stomping grounds at the Fort Wayne Children's Zoo on Zoo Loo Au day, the annual special day for zoo members and their families. As it turned out, this was the last one he would ever attend. The summer was meant for making memories and reliving old memories before he headed back to London that fall.

On a late summer sunny Sunday day in September, Francis left Fort Wayne to fly back to England. Friends from church hosted a backyard cookout with a surprise, impromptu air show put on by some unwitting pilot who was flying in circles by the DeKalb County Airport. Betty and James saw him off at the Fort Wayne airport this time. After a prayerful, uneventful flight, he landed back "home" in London the next morning.

A Harrowing New Bike Route

Honoring the promise he had made to his mother, Francis set about finding himself a used bike to take between his hall and his classrooms instead of using the tube. On the very day he landed, he searched all around until he found a used bike. From that point on, each morning and evening, he rode his bike across busy central London between Russell Square and London Bridge, falling off his bike in busy traffic at least four times in busy traffic, nearly getting run over each time! The truth was he was easily spooked while trying to ride among the buses and lorries and cars, and he believes that once again the LORD's hand was upon him, protecting him from harm in the fast-moving traffic. He certainly did pray!

Unfortunately, Francis had to admit that he was seriously unnerved by the cars, buses, and lorries that rushed by within inches of him, not to mention the constant honking at him as they passed him by. It had gotten to the point where he dreaded the ride every morning. After a particular harrowing ride to class that left him shaken, he decided to find a safer alternative to both the tube and riding his bike. Walking! He didn't waste any time finding several different routes by which he could just walk across the city center from his hall to the London Bridge. "Urban hiking," as he referred to it, quickly became his favorite mode of transportation no matter where he was in the world. Besides, he soon discovered that this was the best way to learn London, or any city for that matter, like the "back of his hand." From the end of the second year through his third and final year, he walked every day to and from class.

Close Encounters of a Cadaverous Kind

Fortunately, Francis was too focused on his second year, which was incorporated of embryology and human anatomy along with other related courses, to pay much attention to his dangerous crossings. He learned the genetic and molecular mechanisms that control the development of particular tissues and organs in embryonic development and how cells influence one another to adopt certain fates to become specific tissues through molecular signaling between cells. Craniofacial development in the embryo was of particular interest to Francis, as was the use of embryos from chickens and mice as models to study embryonic development in the lab. His thorough study of embryology and developmental biology that year built a strong foundation for his future research in craniofacial developmental biology.

No wonder, Betty warned her son to behave around cadavers: human anatomy and his work in the dissection theatre quickly became one of his favorite passions.

The large dissection theatre was located in the basement of one of the oldest buildings at Guy's Hospital—the early nineteenth-century Hodgkin Building. This cavernous room with its frosted glass windows was filled with ranks of metal tables covered with metal coffinlike boxes. Great care and respect was taken when the coffin tables were open. The living and dead introduced themselves to one another. After all, these cadavers were once living beings that selflessly donated their earthly tents to this wonderful learning institution. Some cadavers seemed more at rest than others, and Francis couldn't help his curiosity about their spiritual choices during their time on earth. Around each table were students and a tutor assigned to that particular cadaver for the year. Francis's total lack of a sense of smell was a blessing; the room reeked of formaldehyde. These bodies were embalmed in a special way in order to preserve them long term, unlike the usual embalming done by American funeral homes that go to great lengths to make bodies look presentable to their loved ones for a few days in their caskets. Instead, while these bodies did not look the least bit alive or presentable, they were treated in a way to preserve them for at least the year they were studied. Their arteries and veins were injected with red and blue wax respectively in order to make them distinguishable as such for students to easily identify them. Students embarked on a systematic dissection and study of human anatomy based on each organ system and region of the body. Later that year, he began bringing his sketchbook and pens to the dissection room at the request of his professors who knew of his artistic talents and started drawing the region that was being dissected.

Francis actually had two different anatomy courses that year; the main one focused on the entire body below the head and neck. A separate course that also included dissection focused on the head and neck only. This was in a smaller but just as ancient dissection theatre, where students dissected heads that they removed from the bodies. At the end of the year, many of the students displayed their anatomical sketches in an anatomy department art show, including his. This artistic event was thought of by Francis and his anatomy instructors, and from that point on, the art show became an annual event in the department.

A New Home Church

At last, after nearly one year of trying to find a home church to attend in London, Francis happened to be walking along Tottenham Court Road one Sunday morning. There he saw an old red brick church that was once the church of eighteenth-century evangelist George Whitefield. This church was the home of a congregation called the American Church in London. Intrigued, he walked in and was immediately surrounded by a warm welcoming atmosphere that was in direct contrast to the cool rather impersonal atmospheres of many of the previous churches he had attended. The pastor was an American as this church used American pastors of the Protestant Reformed traditions, and the parishioners were American expats and other expats from other countries. The worship was Reformed traditional; the pastor wore a black robe with a colored sash, and the congregation sang traditional old hymns to the accompaniment of an antique pipe organ and a piano and robed choir.

New visitors were encouraged to stand and introduce themselves at the beginning of service each Sunday, so Francis did so at his first service. Friendships were formed quickly within the congregation, and there was no doubt in his mind that this church was going to be his church home for the duration of his stay. One older gentleman he befriended invited him to join several others for a trip south of London to East Grinstead to visit the Bluebell Railway— the volunteer-run heritage railway—where restored steam locomotives and wooden carriages with compartments were operated and taken on excursions. One cold clear fall day, the group rode on a train hauled by a majestic large green steam engine that once ran the Golden Arrow services back in the thirties and forties. Cozily inside their wood-paneled compartment, they enjoyed the passing verdant scenery and woodlands. From that point on, once a month, he joined a group from church who would take a hike somewhere out in the countryside outside London, where they held an annual picnic in Regents Park.

One wonderful day in 2006, one of the older ladies from his church, Livvy, introduced Francis to a group of her friends. She invited him to her town home in a lovely older section of London, where he met her friends over tea. The ladies' group nicknamed themselves Francis's "harem," and from that point on, they spent many lovely evenings for dinner on a regular basis. The faithful harem looked after him for the rest of his time there. Their friendships were firm, and after he left and returned to the U.S., they all remained in touch.

Embryonic Research

During the summer of 2006, Francis was put in touch with a professor, Dr. Martyn Cobourne, from the craniofacial development department at Guy's Hospital. The purpose was for him to participate in a summer laboratory research project. The department had the entire twenty-seventh and twenty-eighth floors for their lab space.

Together, they wrote up a grant request and submitted their application to the Welcome Trust U.K. for funding. As soon as the funds were awarded, Francis joined the lab for the summer and, together with Dr. Cobourne, experienced his first adventure in craniofacial embryonic development. At last, he quickly discovered that he had found his niche. Their project was to trace the expression pattern of a novel gene, which was important to craniofacial development, in mouse embryos. By extracting the embryos from pregnant mice and preserving them, then making the embryos translucent in clearing agents, they were able to determine the new gene's expression pattern in them. Using the existing DNA of the gene, Francis designed a complementary messenger RNA (mRNA) probe to home in on the presence of the gene's DNA in the embryos. With a dye attached to the probe, he could see where the gene in question was present in the translucent embryos. The gentlemen took photos of the embryos, and along with the data, they were contributed to a paper that was published the next year. As a coauthor, this became Francis's first published scientific paper.

Boeing Boeing—And Then Some

In July of that same year, a church friend gifted Francis with both a press pass and a regular ticket to the international air show at Farnborough, a biannual event that alternated with the Paris Le Bourget air show. There, the major aerospace companies of the world—including

Airbus, Boeing, and some European and Russian firms—introduced their new civilian and military aircraft and technologies to the public and press. Francis was completely enamored with the new Airbus A380 double-decker super-jumbo jet on display and later on watched it do an actual flying demonstration. In the Airbus pavilion, there was a full-scale mock-up of the interior with its ocean liner-esque grand staircase from the main to the upper deck, which was complete with a first-class lounge and bar.

Over at the Boeing pavilion, the new 787 Dreamliner was promoted in a similar fashion, complete with an interior mock-up with a spacey-looking mood lighting and sculpted interior design. Outside, the Russian Air Force demonstrated the MiG-29 Fulcrum fighter jet and its astounding aerobatic capabilities with high-Gs. The Royal Air Force did a heritage flyby using Spitfires from the Battle of Britain and a World War II Lancaster bomber. The U.S., Russian, and European air forces were neck and neck displaying new aircraft and helicopters while the civil aircraft firms brought out their own new passenger jets. Thus, the purpose of the air show: to sell new civil and military aircraft while wowing the public.

Another Narrow Escape

Finally, in mid-August 2006, Francis flew home for a short summer break, his last one before returning to the U.S. permanently. No sooner was he home when the news broke that authorities in London had apprehended a group of terrorists making liquid bombs to use to blow up transatlantic flights going from London to various North American hub cities on the very day he flew home! Once again, he bowed his head in prayer, thanking the LORD for His wonderful protection. This was a narrow escape that sent chills down his spine and sent Betty into apocalyptic meltdown. Thank goodness, his short visit was action-packed, so there was little time to think about what could have been a tragic end. Together with Betty, Ruth, and James, they experienced their last camping trip as a family. At Chain O'Lakes, they enjoyed camping, hiking, and canoeing, simply enjoying their time together. Francis had brought his old bike from home to ride on the camp trails and his guitar. Before long, it was time to return to London for his final school year.

London's Final Year

King's College London was introducing a new craniofacial embryology research program that would intercalate with the normal degree programs of its students, and Francis joined the inaugural group that was initially very small. It was a new curriculum within a curriculum, and its purpose was to introduce craniofacial science in principle and practice, and the students were required to cap it off with a thesis at the end of the year.

The first semester was largely lecture based and involved classes on the scientific basis of craniofacial development in embryos followed by basic laboratory techniques that, thanks to his previous research earlier that summer, Francis was ahead of the game. Students were required to meet with their prospective lab supervising professors to design and write up grant-style research proposals for their individual thesis projects. Together with Dr. "Pip" Francis-West, they hatched a plan to analyze the expression of particular genes that regulate craniofacial muscle development in chicken embryos.

The spring 2007 semester was devoted to Francis's thesis project that he worked on with Pip in her lab. There, he was introduced to the techniques of collecting chick embryos from their eggs, preserving them in formaldehyde-based fixative, and preparing them for gene expression analysis, procedures similar to those he had previously used on the mouse embryos. Additional techniques he learned were to embed the embryos into glycerin cubes and slice them into very thin sections using a mechanical guillotine-type apparatus enabling him to get cross sections and enable deeper gene expression pattern visualization inside the embryos using mRNA probes specific to the genes of interest under the microscope.

Later that spring, Francis presented a poster in a session invigilated by examiners both within King's and from other institutions. One of his external examiners was Dr. Dixon, the doctor who discovered the Treacher Collins syndrome gene. He wrote his thesis based on his data and results from the chick embryonic muscle developmental gene analyses, which was very well received.

Almost to the Finish Line

The spring semester proved to be pivotal for Francis. His work had gained the admiration of his professors who collectively encouraged him to become a PhD himself in the craniofacial embryology research field. Not wasting a moment, he and Pip applied for one in her lab at King's, and he also applied for PhD courses at institutions in Cincinnati, Los Angeles, San Francisco, and Salt Lake City, among others in the U.S. Almost immediately, he was contacted by a professor from the University of Southern California (USC), in Los Angeles, who invited him to interview. No sooner had he accepted the invitation when he was contacted by the University of California San Francisco (UCSF), whose craniofacial department was also interested in him. Killing two birds with one stone, he planned to fly from London to both Los Angeles and San Francisco to interview in one trip. In April 2007, he boarded a British Airways 747 from London to Los Angeles and spent the next day interviewing at the craniofacial research department at USC and its professor and students. The following day, he flew to San Francisco where he attended a Giants baseball game and got a personalized bat! He spent the entire next day with several of the faculty at UCSF's burgeoning craniofacial research division. The first interview was with Dr. John Greenspan, a warm, personable British native and King's alumnus, thus a fellow King's man. Their connection was immediate, and Dr. Greenspan quickly became a father figure to him. He wasted no time at all introducing Francis to a few of the other faculty who had their own labs. He was interviewed by a panel consisting of several of these people along with the department administrators. Exhausted and jet-lagged, he boarded a plane back to London the next day. A few weeks later, he was notified that both USC and UCSF had accepted him into their PhD programs; he had a choice to make. After some personal deliberation, Francis decided on UCSF for its warm and accepting atmosphere and the fact that San Francisco had a far more tolerable climate, not to mention it was a far easier city to navigate on his own than Los Angeles was with its horrid hot smoggy weather and car-dependent sprawling nature. The future Dr. Francis Joel Smith was on his way!

Beam Me Up, Francis!

Before he left London though, Francis had a few more adventures to partake in: a Star Trek convention and a game of cricket. A longtime Trekkie, he attended his first convention in London in 2005 at the Metropole Hotel in Marble Arch. There, he met so many of the illustrious stars, most notably his favorite, Leonard Nimoy who played Mr. Spock. He also met Patrick Stewart who played Captain Jean-Luc Picard and far too many others to list individually. When Nimoy passed away in 2015, Francis's memory of him became more poignant.

The Hallway Cricket Field

While not exactly a sports aficionado, Francis developed a serious curiosity toward cricket, a national obsession in the U.K. Derived from a number of simple folk bat-and-ball-and-target games played by the peasants during the mediaeval era of England, games like rounders, cricket, and eventually the U.S. game of baseball were developed. After reading about the basics of cricket and after watching some TV games, he paid a visit to the museum at the Marylebone Cricket Club. After learning just about everything he possibly could about the game, the one thing he hadn't done was to watch a live game. He wasn't about to leave the U.K. without doing so.

One day after church, Francis walked over to the Lord's Cricket Ground where he watched his first live game between England and the West Indies. From that moment on, he was hooked. That very evening on the way back to his hall, he dropped by a store and purchased his own cricket bat and ball to take home with him. Earlier that spring, he and his hall neighbors engaged in an impromptu cricket match in the basement bar-lounge area, using a homemade cricket bat and an upturned barstool as a wicket. In one innings (both singular and plural), he was the bowler. In the next, he was the batsman. Unlike his previous engagements in sports that usually ended up in disaster, he found he was able to hit the ball a few times partly due to the broad shape of the cricket bat.

I Shall Return

In a blink of an eye, seemingly, Francis's three years in London were coming to a close. To complete his degree program at King's College London, he submitted and defended his thesis, all the while packing up numerous boxes to ship home. To him, it was over as abruptly as it all began. For the last few weeks, he visited his favorite London haunts for the last time. He even flew to Zurich, Switzerland, to attend a plane spotters' meet up he had been invited to. His "harem"—Livvy and the other wonderful ladies who had taken him under their wing—treated him to a wonderful restaurant for his last meal with them. The last few of his days were emotional and heartrending as he bid an emotional farewell to all his dear friends who were far more like family to him. They were heartbroken to see him go, and he was equally heartbroken to leave. Even the head admissions tutor he had first met on his initial visit to King's four years earlier expressed his deep sense of loss at his departure. For his last outing, he was treated to an evening in a nearby pub, the Bunch of Grapes, with Guy's campus chaplains. For his last piano performance in his church, he played "In Paradisum," the haunting final movement of Gabriel Faure's *Requiem* on the church piano, followed by a repeat performance at the Guy's Hospital chapel's antique Bechstein grand piano. It was a very sad "farewell."

Just as Gen. Douglas MacArthur famously promised, "I shall return," Francis swore that he too would someday come back "home" to London. Over the past three years, he had become so deeply rooted in the British culture he could never imagine life again without some future return. No matter where he ended up working, he vowed he would someday return to the "mothership."

As other American expatriates before him, he had experienced what he coined as the "London syndrome" to describe his insatiable desire to return again to London someday. Spending the years there that Francis was able to had irrevocably changed his outlook. Where before he had been a "typical American" in regard to politics and culture, he had experienced far more beyond what he had even dared to hope for. To this day, he credits the LORD for orchestrating his time in London that helped shape him into the well-rounded person he is today. His time there is and always will be one of the richest experiences of his life.

There was no time for Francis to languish in his sadness for too long. He would touch down back home in Fort Wayne, Indiana, for barely a month before needing to go to San Francisco for the next stage of his life—the pursuit of a PhD in craniofacial embryology.

Book 7

For Thou didst form my inward parts;
Thou didst weave me in my mother's womb.
I will give thanks to Thee,
for I am fearfully and wonderfully made;
Wonderful are Thy works,
And my soul knows it very well.

—Psalm 139

Chapter 1

Westward Ho!
2007–2012

O Lord, Thou has searched me and known me.
Thou dost know when I sit down
and when I rise up;
Thou dost understand my thoughts from afar.
Thou dost scrutinize my path
and my lying down,
And art intimately acquainted
with all my ways.
Even before there is a word on my tongue,
Behold, O Lord, Thou dost know it all.
Thou hast enclosed me behind and before,
And laid Thy hand upon me.
Such knowledge is too wonderful for me;
It is too high, I cannot attain to it.

—Psalm 139:1–6

Tying Up the Loose Ends

Francis's month-long visit home in Fort Wayne passed by like a tornado in full spin. The joy he felt in knowing he was, at last, in the LORD's perfect will for his life engulfed him in indescribable peace. Literally, he could feel God's omniscience and omnipresence in every passing moment. He couldn't help but marvel at the intimate way in which God was acquainted with him. No matter where he was, whether at rest or at play, God always knew his motives and thoughts before he clothed them in words. There is absolutely nothing the LORD didn't know about him! What a wonderful thought. Between visiting family and old friends and unpacking his numerous boxes from London only to repack new boxes for San Francisco, there wasn't any down time. His scheduled arrival date at the University of California San Francisco was barely one month away.

On top of it all and of utmost personal importance, Francis had scheduled a visit to the Children's Craniofacial Association (CCA) annual Cher's Family Retreat. The retreat had been something he dearly missed while he was in London for three years, and he couldn't wait to be back. That particular year, CCA's retreat was held in Salt Lake City, Utah. He brought along his green violin, which he played for everyone. There were numerous old friends to catch up with and many new people he couldn't wait to get acquainted with. So many of the younger ones he had known when they were mere children were now grown, and many of them were college age and facing the extraordinary excitement of their futures just as he was. Those special two days were jam-packed with visits to a Western town and a theme park outside Salt Lake City and to the temple complex in downtown Salt Lake City. While ambling along in downtown, Francis suffered sunstroke in the brutal sun, and when the group got back to the hotel, he had to be cooled down by wrapping cold wet towels around his head. For the last evening there, the group enjoyed a family-style dinner, and during that time, Francis delighted in dancing with the ladies. After such a long absence, this was one of the most enjoyable retreats he had been on, and he vowed that he would never again go for such a lengthy time without reconnecting with this special community he loved so much. From that point on, he attended the CCA retreat on a regular basis.

Meanwhile, Back at the Funeral Home

Sometime during this summertime break, Betty decided it was time to sell their beloved Garrett home. She and Ruth were alone now, and they could no longer manage such a large house by themselves, where the achingly empty rooms were as silent as tombs. Even her thoughts seemed to echo throughout the house. Ruth and Francis stepped up to the plate, and the three of them painted the inside and the outside of the house. Years earlier, Ruth and Francis meticulously laid new flooring in the front rooms and refinished the parlor's hardwood floor, pretty much on their own, which was no easy feat, and now they got busy to make it look like new again. The Smiths had owned the large home on "Harrison Hill" (as they called it since it was on a hill along Harrison Street) since 1979—twenty-eight years! Hanging on the old lamppost on the front lawn that once held the Baidinger-Walter Funeral Home sign was a "For Sale" sign that, for them, was painful to even look at. Even more daunting was now Betty had to house hunt.

With the goal of finding a single-story home, Betty, Francis, and Ruth charged all over Fort Wayne, Allen County, and DeKalb County. Near Red Cedar Center, where Ruth had once learned to ride horseback, they looked at a country house with a lake. But alas, it was too expensive. They looked at another semirural house north of Fort Wayne. Outside Auburn, they looked at two other country houses. Not finding anything that suited Betty's needs, it was decided that her best bet would for her to be in the city proper. Fort Wayne provided a far broader spectrum of houses, not to mention everything Betty needed would be within easy reach. For several days, the group plus their realtor explored numerous ideal candidates for Betty's new home.

San Francisco, Here We Come!

By this time, Francis was doing some home hunting of his own. After searching for and discovering that he could not possibly afford private sector housing due to the stratospheric rents, he focused on the university's new high-rise student apartment housing estate at their newest campus in downtown San Francisco. The campus had four towering blocks of flats, in ascending order of height. A studio flat would suffice for his minimal needs. He settled on a three-hundred-seventy-nine-square-foot unit with a kitchen as well as a bathroom. It was the least expensive option he could find. After his application was approved, he was given a move-in date of July 20.

Between Betty's house hunting, CCA, fixing up the house, visiting with family and friends, and unpacking and repacking, Francis was exhausted. He had to go through a lifetime of belongings, getting rid of what he no longer needed, which was mostly books, and packing up kitchenware, cutlery, dishes, and other household and personal necessities and clothes that temporarily had to be stored in his bedroom. Of course, his green violin, acoustic guitar, and an antique trombone that was a family heirloom he was taking along. His piano, which was too big to move, had to stay behind. He also had to pack childhood mementos, his personal medical collection, and his favorite airplane models and toys, among other stuff. While packing up his artwork, he left out a few favored drawings for Betty to take to her new house, most notably his India-ink painting of a grand piano at IPFW, which was one of her favorites. Francis even had to pack furniture with him in order to fill up his small studio apartment. He packed a small bedside table that Bob had made decades ago, his green La-Z-Boy, a dresser, and a twin mattress and bed frame. To avoid many of the moving costs, he and Ruth arranged to convoy it across the United States with his boxes packed in his

Pontiac sedan and his furniture packed under a tarp in her Dodge pickup truck.

The Great San Francisco Earthquake

Moving day arrived on a hot and sticky mid-July day. After several days of farewells, Francis and Ruth were ready to hit the road for the long trek across country to the City by the Bay. Fortunately, Ruth had the foresight to bring their niece, Meg, along for help and companionship. They pushed out of Garrett as the sun was setting in a two-car convoy reminiscent of a scene from *Grapes of Wrath* by John Steinbeck. They crossed Indiana on US 30 to Chicago, where they got on Interstate 80 for the long haul westward. Hitting a midwest thunderstorm, they spent the first road night in an Econo Lodge, in Princeton, Illinois. Over the next few days—barely stopping each night to sleep in a motel or rest area—they hauled through Illinois, Iowa, and Nebraska, then onto Wyoming and Utah where they drove through the most desolate alien landscape he had ever seen: the Bonneville Salt Flats. While at a rest stop, Francis used a shot glass to scoop up some salt, a souvenir he still has. After catching a brief rest, the trio trekked through Nevada and, at last, onto Northern California!

After slogging through the San Francisco rush-hour traffic, they arrived at Francis's new home, just before sundown. His tower block was in the China Basin area that had once been warehouses. After retrieving the keys to his apartment and copies of his lease documents, the trio moved everything from their two vehicles into his new third-floor apartment. The tower was built like a fortress from reinforced concrete that looked strong enough to withstand any earthquake that was a constant threat in the Bay Area. Francis could not have been more pleased with the stark white simplicity of his new apartment; it was stunning. A wide floor-to-ceiling glass window with views of the new San Francisco Giants baseball stadium and the downtown skyline adorned the north side of the apartment while, on the east-facing side, the windows were vertical slits. Black granite countertops adorned the kitchen and bathroom countertops. Inside the kitchen were a full-sized stove, oven, and dishwasher; but the one oddity was the refrigerator was only waist-high with a small freezer shelf. The assumption was college students probably didn't cook much, but obviously, they didn't know Francis. He had planned all along to do all his own cooking. The apartment was about the size of a cruise ship stateroom, but it was perfect for his needs. Since Francis had just moved in, there was no food, so the group had to dine out for the evening at the nearest local KFC franchise! The next day, they explored some downtown sights and ate at a chrome diner. Once Francis was happily ensconced in his new apartment, Ruth and Meg headed back home to Indiana.

An Academic Research Plan

Within a few more days, Francis began his studies in earnest at UCSF. During a meeting with his advisors whom he had previously met during his interview that spring, an academic and research plan was designed for both the near future and long-term future. Although it was still midsummer, he was set up for the first of three semester-length laboratory rotations, whose purpose was to introduce him to the research in three different mentors' labs, each of which had a different project in progress. Francis's first lab rotation was in Dr. Ramos's lab. Dr. Ramos was researching the interaction of oral squamous cell carcinoma cells versus normal oral tissue cells, with the extracellular matrix or scaffolding. He was introduced to cell culture methods under conditions almost as sterile as an operating theater, fluorescent cell staining, and fluorescent microscopy as methods for observing cancer cells' interaction with the surrounding scaffolding. Under the microscope, the molecules for which he was staining the cell cultures showed up fluorescent green. The images were so beautiful and fascinating that Francis actually considered having some of them framed to hang on his wall as art pieces.

Dr. Ramos and Francis became fast friends, both of whom were huge baseball fans. Together, they took every opportunity to attend as many home Giants games as possible. After all, the stadium was a short walkable distance from his Mission Bay apartment. Much to Dr. Ramos's chagrin, he discovered his charge was a die-hard St. Louis Cardinals fan, but Francis soon made room in his heart for the Giants. Dr. Ramos rejoiced!

Encouraging Others

Nothing is more important for Francis than his God-given desire to encourage others who suffer from craniofacial anomalies. No sooner had he come to know his professors and peers at UCSF when he became aware of a family whose young daughter had Treacher Collins syndrome, and they were all struggling. In spite of his busy schedule, Francis decided to take a weekend off to visit the family in Maryland. Upon landing in Baltimore, he rented a Chrysler PT Cruiser convertible and drove to Salisbury to visit the family. The visit, although short, was fruitful. Francis and the family spent a good time of witnessing, fellowship, and encouragement. The family was extremely grateful for the gift of a new outlook in place of despair that only someone who had suffered as they had could give them. To Francis, he was simply doing what the LORD assigned him to do, and the outcome was always to the glory of the LORD.

Betty's Great San Francisco Adventure

As a surprise to Betty for her birthday in late September, family and friends gathered together to buy her an airplane ticket to fly out to San Francisco to see her son. She arrived on a Thursday evening, and from that point on, her visit was nonstop motion trying to keep up with her hyper son. During a visit to the lab where she met Dr. Ramos, Betty got to see one of Francis's slides under a microscope.

From there, she and Francis were off on a tour of San Francisco, slam-bang Francis style. They rode the cable cars to Chinatown where they ate a fabulous Chinese meal in a geisha-style booth, then roamed all over Chinatown on foot, visiting its numerous shops and antique shops.

Chinatown was hilly and overcrowded with pushy people, and trying to keep up with Francis was difficult. "We walked all over," recalled Betty. Along the way, Betty looked longingly at the colorful rickshaws that passed them by, but she couldn't talk Francis into riding in one. "He said the rickshaw took longer than walking, so he wouldn't ride in one. I was exhausted!" Like it or not, she had no other choice but to stay as close to Francis as her aching legs would allow.

The last shop they visited was an antique store where an antique green grand piano was displayed. Francis was not the least bit shy in letting the shop owner know that he was an accomplished pianist. Graciously, the owner extended the invitation for him to sit down and play it. Betty was thankful, not so much for the musical interlude but for the opportunity to rest and get off her legs for a few moments that by now felt like jelly.

All too soon, the short interlude came to an end. Without wasting a beat, they headed to IKEA in Palo Alto where they browsed the never-ending showroom. Francis picked up a rolling island for his kitchen as well as a few other odds and ends he needed for his apartment.

On Saturday morning, the duo engaged in another partial day of sightseeing before eventually ending up at the Giants ballpark for a game that evening, which Betty thoroughly enjoyed. Francis, for whatever reason, decided he wanted to climb to the top of the stadium, with Betty dragging behind him. About halfway up, Betty noticed an elevator that others were riding to the top, and she mentioned it to her son.

"Oh, we don't want to take that," he replied. That was that, and they kept on climbing. Betty not only made it to the top, she somehow managed to make it all the way back down. So this became the fitting end to Betty's whirlwind tour of the City by the Bay, an event she fondly talks about to this day.

Early Sunday morning, Francis drove his exhausted mother to the airport where he bid her adieu. As tired as she was, her visit with her son and his new home remains one of her happiest and most memorable birthdays ever. "I had such a wonderful time," she said.

A Church Family for Francis

Where can I go from Thy Spirit?
Or where can I flee from Thy presence?
If I ascend to heaven, Thou art there;
If I make my bed in Sheol,
behold, Thou art there.
If I take the wings of the dawn,
If I dwell in the remotest part of the sea,
Even there Thy hand will lead me,
And Thy right hand will lay hold of me.

If I say, "Surely the darkness will overwhelm me,
And the light around me will be night,"
Even the darkness is not dark to Thee,
And the night is as bright as the day.
Darkness and light are alike to Thee.

—Psalm 139:7–12

For Francis though, there was no "rest," a word that seemingly does not exist in his personal vocabulary. The fall semester started off like gangbusters, yet he was constantly motivated by God's presence. No matter what the day brought, he stayed in the Word on a daily basis, and as a result, he exercised caution and discretion so he could spend and use his time wisely. Being in a doctoral program meant a workload like he had never before experienced, yet he was able to run the course in complete confidence. The fall and spring semesters were packed with lecture courses covering cell biology, craniofacial development in embryos, genetics, craniofacial disorders and their treatment, stem cells, and other topics relevant to his research. One of his favorite classes was on craniofacial disorders, aimed mainly at dental students, for it gave Francis a special opportunity to contribute his unique perspective to the class as someone with an actual craniofacial condition.

In order for Francis to feel truly at home in his new life in San Francisco, his immediate desire was to find himself a Bible-preaching, Bible-teaching, Bible-walking church. Finally, he found one near downtown. The services were modern, and the building was filled with happy-clappy music played by a stage band made up of acoustic and electric guitars and percussion. The huge pipe organ, it appeared, was never used, at least not while he was there. Francis attended Sunday morning services for several weeks, but as much as he loved the people, a voice inside told him he needed to keep on looking.

Francis's efforts soon bore fruit. In March 2008, Francis was led to his new church home. Hamilton Square Baptist Church, located in the heart of downtown, just off Van Ness Avenue at Franklin and Geary, was housed in a lovely 1948 Spanish-style building. The services were traditional with the congregation singing from hymnals, accompanied by a grand piano and organ along with a robed choir, which he dearly loved. The building's design, inside and out, reminded him a bit of Europe, which suited him since he was still homesick for London. He quickly came to think of this church as his "Baptist Cathedral" as its majestic design was peculiar to the Baptist churches he was used to. Its pastor, Dr. Pastor David Innes, a chipper fellow who was of Scottish descent, loved the LORD with his entire being, and it showed. Pastor Innes's preaching style was more like teaching as he gave detailed exposition of Bible passages with his wonderful delivery and sense of humor. For a short while, Francis attended both churches, one in the morning and Hamilton in the evening. Soon though, he started attending both services at Hamilton. From the first evening he attended at Hamilton, people reached out to him in genuine warmth. It didn't take long for him to join the music ministry where he started playing solos for the offertory on either his green violin or the grand piano.

Before long, he went on a singles ministry retreat at a Christian retreat center that resembled a castle. Hamilton Square Baptist Church was his home church for the next four years (and remains to this day his number one priority to visit whenever he's back in town).

Betty's New Home

In April, Francis received the wonderful news that Betty had finally found her new home in Fort Wayne after nearly one year of house hunting. Ruth broke the news to him with photos of it. It was a midfifties ranch located in a subdivision not five minutes east of IPFW in an area rich with supermarkets, a veterinary clinic, gas stations, and other conveniences easily reached by a brief drive. The Garrett home was sold to an attorney with a huge family, and from the proceeds, she was able to purchase her new home. Friends and family gathered together to help with the move.

That summer, Francis got to visit Betty and Ruth's new home. Betty still had her favorite pieces of his artwork framed and hanging on the walls among the numerous other mementos of her many children she loved to display for everyone to see. A ramp had been built inside the garage to enable Ruth to maneuver her wheelchair in and out of the house. The kitchen was painted in a cheerful fifties red-and-black scheme, complete with retro Coca-

Cola ads on the kitchen walls. Both the kitchen and dining room overlooked an expansive backyard with an above-ground pool. It was a great place for the dogs to run and for Betty and Ruth to garden in. It even had a small storage barn. There were three large bedrooms, one of which became Francis's *de facto* bedroom for when he came for a visit. In the front was a lovely family room, complete with a stone fireplace flanked by bookshelves, a style popular in the fifties. The neighborhood was a clean, quiet one, an older subdivision full of similar vintage houses. All in all, it was affordable and manageable for Betty, instead of being so far away in Garrett as the other house was. The visit was a short one, but Francis was very pleased with his mother's new home.

Chapter 2

The Mad Scientist

For Thou didst form my inward parts;
Thou didst weave me in my mother's womb.
I will give thanks to Thee,
for I am fearfully and wonderfully made;
Wonderful are Thy works,
And my soul knows it very well.
My frame was not hidden from Thee,
When I was made in secret,
And skillfully wrought in the depths of the earth.
Thine eyes have seen my unformed substance;
And in Thy book they were all written,
The days that were ordained for me,
When as yet there was not one of them.
                        —Psalm 139:13–16

Among Francis's favorite Bible verses were Psalms 139:13–16, which touched his life enormously, obviously on an extremely personal basis. As he and Dr. Marcucio created a project together to observe the effects of early embryonic hypoxia (oxygen deprivation) on craniofacial development, he often thought of these particular verses that acknowledge God's power to create human life: "Thou didst weave..."

How marvelous for Francis that his life was so important to his LORD that through his own craniofacial maladies, he was going to be used mightily to not only help others who had been afflicted as he had; he was also going to be a witness to all for what the LORD had done in his own life. For God is not only the Creator; He has divine purpose in all things. Francis was constantly amazed to where he was being led and how through his craniofacial research he was going to be a blessing to so many others who had been afflicted with craniofacial anomalies. After all, it is through trials and difficulties that people turn to and cling to the LORD. It is human nature that when life is going well, there is little perception for their own need for God. What many people consider a challenge, God would use as blessings for His glory. Every single life is important to God.

Quicks, Qucks, and Duails

When Francis returned to San Francisco that summer, an exciting new project in another lab was waiting for him. Dr. Marcucio, his new mentor, specialized in both orthopedic trauma research and craniofacial embryonic development. Besides, he had his own large lab on the beautiful historic campus of San Francisco General Hospital in the Potrero district in southern San Francisco. With Dr. Marcucio, all their work would be with chick embryos *in ovo*.

To mimic hypoxia, they devised an incubator with a nitrogen gas supply and an oxygen sensor/controller to lower the interior oxygen level in the chamber by pumping nitrogen into it. After incubating the eggs for several days, they removed the embryos and observed them for cranio-facial malformations. Many of the embryos did not survive the oxygen deprivation, and those that did were smaller and had a variety of craniofacial deformities ranging from a simple lack of symmetry to gross defects, including missing facial features or no face at all, and exposed or missing brains. Then he took images of these embryos under a microscope. He embedded many of them in wax, sliced them into thin sections, and stained them for microscopic analysis of their tissues and cells. Unfortunately, his summer lab rotation ended before his hypoxia research was complete, but he planned to return to it later on. Francis did, however, present his preliminary results, which were quite promising, at a school-wide research event that fall, where he earned first prize for his talk.

The next academic year was focused mostly on research rather than classes. Francis's third rotation was spent with Dr. Schneider whose lab was on the main campus. His lab specialized in bird skull development, working with chick, duck, and quail embryos. Francis's project was to compare jaw development between duck and quail embryos. For this, Dr. Schneider introduced him to his pioneering technique of creating a hybrid quail-duck embryo called a "quck" in which a piece of the quail embryonic head was grafted onto a duck embryo head and allowed to develop. After incubating the duck eggs for a certain amount of time after this chimeric surgery on the embryos, he removed the resulting quck embryos and observed whether there was a difference in the rate of jaw development between the two species. In another project, he treated some quail and duck eggs with drugs that affected bone development. He took quck, quail, and duck embryos and embedded them in wax and sliced them in thin sections for microscopic analysis of their jaw tissues in order to compare development between species under certain conditions. Eventually, he came to the conclusion that not only qucks could be generated by creation of hybrid bird embryos but other combinations of bird species were plausible, such as quail to chick (quick) and duck to quail (duail). From that point on, Francis deemed himself "the Mad Scientist."

International Conferences

Sometime during the spring 2009 semester, Dr. Ramos encouraged Francis to attend an international dental conference in Miami in March. Although he did not present, he was able to meet many other potential colleagues and attend interesting research and clinical sessions during his week in Miami, along with enjoying the beaches and the Art Deco architecture of the hotels and restaurants in the area.

At the meeting in Miami, Francis attended a gathering of his UCSF colleagues one evening at another hotel where he networked with some professors from New Zealand. While discussing his ongoing hypoxia research in chick embryos, Francis was extended an invitation for him to speak at a future meeting at their dental school in New Zealand.

Two weeks later, Francis was invited to attend and present his own research at an international anatomy meeting in New Orleans, which he gratefully accepted. In a cavernous conference center, he presented a poster he created with the results (to date) of his work with hypoxic chick embryos, which garnered a great deal of interest from others. Francis also received quite a surprise: also in attendance were his former anatomy professors from King's College! Francis and the ladies wasted no time in engaging in something fun together, a lunch cruise on a steamboat along the riverfront in New Orleans.

In July, Francis presented at his third international conference, this time right at home in San Francisco. To a global audience of leading researchers in developmental biology, he offered his poster again. By attending these conferences, he was able to share his up-and-coming research with his colleagues and learn from theirs. Assuredly, along with building his own professional reputation while connecting with others in the field worldwide, he was gaining future job opportunities.

Meanwhile, Francis rejoined Dr. Marcucio's lab because he was convinced that the chick hypoxia work they had previously started held great promise and should be continued. There was a need to expand beyond observation of the various craniofacial malformations in chick embryos starved of oxygen and dig deeper to the levels of cellular and molecular responses to oxygen deprivation to better understand why the defects were occurring. Francis then decided to pursue this further as the topic for his doctoral dissertation, and from that point, he dug in his heels for the next four years of hard work.

More Profound Adventures

While continuing his experiments with hypoxic chick embryos in order to gather more preliminary data and evidence, Francis began writing his research proposal describing additional experiments that should be done and their predicted results. His proposal was to observe the effects of different amounts of oxygen below normal, from mild to very severe hypoxia and for various periods of time, compared to normal oxygen conditions. He devised experiments that would measure the proliferation and death of cells in hypoxic versus normal embryos along with the plan to measure particular molecular responses to hypoxia. The research proposal consisted of a background "story" describing craniofacial anomalies in embryos and preliminary data he had collected up-to-date on the hypoxic chick embryos as well as proposed experiments and the rationale for them and what the expected outcomes of those studies were going to be. The proposal was written in research grant proposal form that scientists normally wrote to agencies such as the National Institutes of Health (NIH), the major U.S. government research grant funding agency supporting most of the nation's scientific and medical research.

At last, it was time for Francis to prepare for his qualifying exam that would officially deem him as a doctoral candidate. For this exam, he gathered a committee of examiners consisting of Dr. Marcucio and other professors under him whom he had been working with in the craniofacial PhD program at UCSF. Collectively, they helped him write his research proposal and had periodic meetings with him in order to help him prepare for the exam. The format of the exam comprised both an oral defense and a written exam based on not only the proposal itself but more of his accumulated knowledge of craniofacial embryonic development. In February 2010, after he submitted his proposal to the committee and the department, he took the comprehensive written exam in a quiet room, alone. The answers were in essay form, and he drew pictures and diagrams to support his answers. During the oral session, he answered a myriad of questions the committee fired at him, in increasing order of complexity. After the oral exam, his panel deliberated for a bit, then called him back into their room to congratulate him on passing the qualifying exam, which officially made him a PhD candidate free to go on with his proposed research. Francis couldn't wait to call Betty and tell her the wonderful news

A Kiwi Welcome

How precious also are Thy thoughts to me, O God!
If I should count them, they would outnumber the sand.
When I awake, I am still with Thee!
—Psalm 139:17–18

Around that time same time, Francis received an official invitation from his colleagues in New Zealand to be a keynote lecturer for their Research Day at the University of Otago in Dunedin in April 2010. Immediately, his thoughts and prayers turned to preparing for a lecture on embryo hypoxia research along with a talk about his own unique life experience connected to his craniofacial research career. Each and every step of the way, he was constantly amazed at the doors that the LORD was opening for him. Just before Palm Sunday, he boarded the first of three flights it would take to deliver him to Dunedin, located at the south end of the South Island. In the over twenty-four hours of flight, he crossed the International Date Line, and he went from springtime to fall. He was truly "down under." Even his colorful vivid dreams of his upcoming trip did not compare to the splendorous reality of the adventure he was about to face. Stepping off the plane, he received a Kiwi welcome (a very warm welcome from New Zealand people who are known as Kiwis) from the immigration officer at Auckland airport to the female chauffeur driver of the Jaguar who picked him up at the airport to deliver him to the university's own hotel.

Planes, Trains, and Automobiles

After a brief, albeit jet-lagged, rest, Francis visited the dental school and spent time with the professors who had invited him where they got to know one another. The first half of the day was spent at the orthodontics clinic where the gentleman in charge took him to lunch nearby. Although his hosts encouraged him to get out and explore Dunedin and the central Otago region, he certainly didn't need any prodding. The city's railway station, much to his delightful surprise, was a Victorian architectural master-piece. For an entire day, he happily rode a vintage train of wooden carriages pulled by an old diesel locomotive, tour-ing all over the Taieri Gorge, a mountainous area. The train took him through tunnels in mountains and over trestle bridges through valleys, sheep pastures, and wine country, then stopping for a couple of breaks for its passengers to enjoy the majestic scenery.

The time Francis was afforded in Dunedin allowed him to explore the small city where he enjoyed the architecture of the Anglican cathedral and some of the churches, uni-versity campus, as well as the more unique modern styles of some buildings and enjoying some of the local restau-rants, not to mention taking photos galore.

The University of Otago Faculty of Dentistry Research Day took place on April 1. Its purpose was to provide an opportunity for the entire dental school community to gather and hear about the latest research and clinical advances in dentistry, oral biology, and craniofacial biology from students, faculty, and guest speakers. Francis was the second of the keynote speakers to speak. During his talk, he first presented an image of himself at three years old, showing his full-blown Treacher Collins syndrome under his then-fiery red hair. The audience was captivated by his life's journey and its connection to his craniofacial research as well as his educational journeys in the US, London, and finally at UCSF. The rest of the talk focused on his latest findings on the effects of embryonic oxygen deprivation on chick craniofacial development. Later on that day, he was able to enjoy the company of his colleagues from Australia, New Zealand, and Asia. That evening, his hosts took him to dinner at a local restaurant where he enjoyed the locally sourced rack of lamb.

The next day was Good Friday, a deeply moving holiday for Christians as it commemorates the crucifixion of Jesus Christ at Calvary. This was also to be Francis's last full day in New Zealand. His heart was full as he thought of Jesus dying on the cross and shedding His own blood so that he might have eternal life. He was also wistful about leaving, for he had had a most memorable time among the warmest people on earth, not to mention the most beautiful scenery imaginable. He didn't want to leave, and he vowed, then and there, to return someday. On Good Friday, he attended a deeply touching commemorative service at the Anglican cathedral on the Octagon, the city's center. Deeply humbled from the moving service and with tremendously mixed feelings, he wandered through the city where he stumbled upon Baldwin Street, the steepest street in the world, pitched at a forty-five-degree grade. Aside from the enormous workout he got, he found the apparent "lean" of the houses an artistic fascination. The steepest streets of San Francisco he was accustomed to, most notably Lombard Street, were nowhere near the steepness of Baldwin Street.

At the crack of dawn the next morning, Francis struggled to wake up for his flight that would take him from Dunedin to Auckland where he was to connect to a Qantas 747 flight back to Los Angeles then onto San Francisco. Oh, how he hated to leave. This was to be another twenty-four-hour trek across the Pacific, where once again he would cross the International Date Line that would put him back into Friday; he was going to gain back that day he lost on the way over! When he touched down in Los Angeles, he was inexplicably blindsided by the worst case of jet lag he ever remembered. He barely recalled the last leg home to San Francisco, but when he finally walked into his apartment, he literally collapsed on his bed where he swears he didn't move for an entire weekend. On Monday, finally refreshed from the "lost weekend," his mind was alive with some of the most marvelous, memorable experiences of his entire lifetime. He remembered each and every face of every person he encountered and every detail of his incredible countryside adventure. This visit was so special to him he was literally already planning for his next one. Except next time, he would include Australia, just one more childhood dream that he knew he would someday visit.

Dr. Frankenstein, I Presume?

With two major accomplishments completed, the qualifying exam and the New Zealand trip, Francis had to snap out of his reverie and get back to work. Right away, he expanded the range of hypoxic oxygen levels from mild to severe to see whether the mortality and incidence of craniofacial anomalies would increase by the lower oxygen levels. While observing the level of cell proliferation with a dye he injected into the embryos that marked cells that were growing and dividing, and after he collected the embryos and looking at slices of their tissues to see how much dye was present, he was able to compare the levels of cell death between normal versus hypoxic embryos with a stain that collected in dead cells. From that procedure, he was able to see an increase in the number of dead embryos after decreasing oxygen levels. Also, he was looking at a possible metabolic stress response in these cells because the oxygen starvation was causing metabolic stress leading to an increase of cell death. From there, he started measuring the change in shape of oxygen-deprived embryos compared to normal ones.

Francis was now able to form a dissertation committee consisting of Dr. Marcucio and others who would oversee and guide his progress over the next three years as his ongoing research allowed him to develop theories to explain his results. The committee met on a regular basis as he presented his ongoing results and possible reasons and theories for them. Through their suggestions, he was able to increase the variety of experiments to test his evolving theories, enabling him to develop as an independent researcher who was constantly coming up with more possible explanations and finding different ways to test his new theories.

All the while, Francis was deep in thought and praying for guidance in order to write his book-length synopsis of the background for his research and rationale, along with his growing amount of data, as well as a discussion explaining the phenomena he was observing.

Canada—A Lasting Impression

That October, Francis took a month-long sabbatical to work in the laboratory at the University of Calgary in Canada, with one of Dr. Marcucio's colleagues, Dr. Benedikt Hallgrimsson. From previous visits, Dr. Hallgrimsson had been able to observe his work in Dr. Marcucio's lab. When he observed Francis doing two-dimensional shape change analysis with the hypoxic and normal chick embryos, he was impressed with his quality of his work and invited him to visit his Calgary lab to work with him and to learn new techniques that would be helpful for his own future research. Under Dr. Hallgrimsson's guidance, he learned to scan the heads of duck and quail embryos in a micro-CT scanner, a smaller version of the CT scanners normally found in hospitals. From those scans, three-dimensional computer images were created, on which Francis placed landmarks, between which he could measure the distance and thereby measure the variation in 3-D craniofacial shape among embryos and between species.

One surprise Francis wasn't expecting was Cher was in town. Somehow, through the grapevine, she learned that Francis was there too. Opening up his e-mail, he was quite surprised to find a personal invitation from her to attend her world tour concert in Calgary and visit him backstage afterward. Going by himself certainly didn't daunt him. Francis felt great warmth for her and all she had done for those who suffered from craniofacial anomalies as he watched her magnificent costume-studded performance from one of the best seats in the house. No sooner had she taken her last bow when someone from her entourage approached him and led him backstage. Greeting each other like old friends, Francis was overwhelmed by her thoughtfulness for thinking of him and his gratitude toward her.

***

While working in the lab, Francis met Dr. Hallgrimsson's postdoctoral fellows and students who worked with him on his sabbatical project. For the duration of his visit, he stayed at the university hotel. Other campus facilities, he discovered, had been used for some of the events in the Winter Olympics in 1988. During his somewhat-limited free time, he explored as much of Calgary that he could pack in. In less than one week after his arrival, he experienced an early snowfall—in October, no less! Calgary, he discovered, was a chilly place; consequently, the skies were gloomy and gray with a few scattered days of sunshine thrown in. Finding a church was always of utmost importance to him, and soon he was led to Northside Baptist Church, pastored by Pastor David Adkins, which was a small church with a warm and loving congregation located inside a Rotary Club building out near Calgary's airport, where he quickly gained a church family. His new friends, derived from both the university and his church, introduced him to the Canadian Thanksgiving, which occurs on the second Monday in October but otherwise very similar to the American one. All too quickly, this fabulous learning adventure came to a close.

Let the message of Christ dwell among you richly
as you teach and admonish one another with all wisdom
through psalms, hymns, and songs from the Spirit,
singing to God with gratitude in your hearts.
—Colossians 3:16

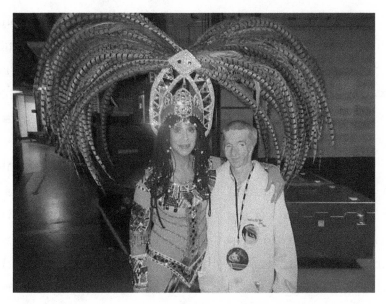

A surprise from Cher

Francis was touched by Cher's thoughtfulness and considers her outreach to those in the craniofacial community to be a shared passion.

Homerun

O That thou wouldst slay the wicked, O God;
Depart from me, therefore, men of bloodshed.
For they speak against Thee wickedly,
and Thine enemies take Thy name in vain.
Do I not hate those who hate Thee, O Lord?
And do I not loathe those who rise up against Thee?
I hate them with the utmost hatred;
They have become my enemies.

—Psalm 139:19–22

In April 2011, Francis attended his second anatomy conference in Washington DC, where he spoke on his findings from his chick research. This was the first time he had given an oral presentation at a major international conference. At his previous conferences, he had always presented his research in the form of a poster.

That next June, Francis was given the opportunity to speak at the annual meeting of the Canadian Hard of Hearing Association (CHHA) in Yellowknife, in the Northwest Territories, which was very close to the Arctic Circle. Surprisingly, the invitation had come from Bill Adkins, the father of Pastor David Adkins who pastored Northside Baptist Church, the church he had attended during his stay in Calgary. Since he was giving the keynote talk, the organization was kind enough to pick up his travel and lodging expenses. No sooner had he landed in Edmonton, Alberta, where he had a long layover, he hit the ground running to explore the antique stores in Old Strathcona, a historic district of Edmonton. He was so caught up in his glorious antiquing adventure he barely made it back to the airport in time to board the flight to Yellowknife. The airport at Yellowknife was so tiny it only had one gate. By comparison, the Fort Wayne airport appeared quite large. As soon as the aircraft door opened and the portable stairs were pushed up against the fuselage of the Boeing 737, Francis became completely disoriented; it was nine thirty at night, and it was broad daylight outside! In the near-arctic summer, the sun does not set at all; it is twenty-four hours of nonstop daylight. It took him a moment to gather his senses before he headed toward the gate area to meet Mr. Adkins who was kind enough to greet him himself. From there, they proceeded to the home of a friend where Francis was to stay for the night.

The next few days were action-packed with exploring and attending the conference where Francis gave his keynote talk on his life without ears, his modern hearing aids, and experiences in dealing with his craniofacial anomalies to a very appreciative audience. He had such an enjoyable visit he found it difficult to board the homeward-bound jet to go home.

***

Back in the lab in San Francisco, Francis began writing his dissertation, which, for all intents and purposes, took the same amount of time as writing a book while continuing on with his experiments. This process took up his entire final year at UCSF. While continuing on with the additional experiments he needed, he also wrote the background (discussion of how craniofacial development occurs by way of the cranial neural crest cells, the progenitors of the craniofacial skeleton and tissues) and rationale for his work. Included was a description of the experiments he had been doing and the results to date. Later, as the experiments came to a conclusion and he had all the data he needed, he began to write up the discussion of the results and their implications for the future and whatever else he believed could be done.

Meanwhile, Francis began looking for postdoctoral fellowships in other craniofacial laboratories including one in New York City and others across the country and across the pond as well as in Canada. He even put his feelers out at his old alma mater in London. It wasn't long before Dr. Hallgrimsson offered him a postdoctoral research fellowship position at the University of Calgary. Dr. Hallgrimsson had observed his morphometrics work he had done over the years. Francis accepted his offer, and he began making preparations for life outside of the United States for the second time, the first being London. Once again, he jumped through all the required hoops, renewing his passport and acquiring a work visa from Canada. Francis had to do a great deal of thinking about how he was going to move up there. There were several options: hiring a moving van on a meager budget, getting rid of almost everything he owned and selling his car versus leaving everything behind in storage. He opted for the storage unit as his car was a necessity in Canada. Whatever he was not able to pack into his Pontiac Bonneville was either donated away or put in storage. There really wasn't much he could pack inside a sedan.

Sadly, he had to miss the June 2012 CCA retreat due to a lack of funds and the burden of finishing the last of his work. But there would be others, he knew. However, that June, Betty and Ruth drove out from Fort Wayne for a week visit, one last time, as he would not complete his work until later that summer, in August. They spent their time driving north, across the Golden Gate Bridge, into Sonoma and

Napa Valley wine country for a day among the vineyards and wineries. Betty visited the lab and met Dr. Marcucio and the rest of his lab colleagues. On Wednesday evening, they attended the evening service at Hamilton Square Baptist Church. On the last day of their visit, they went to Fisherman's Wharf and Pier 39 where they had dinner at Bubba Gump's Shrimp Company restaurant. Their time together was wonderful. For a gift, Francis bought both his sister and mother pilsner glasses with the Bubba Gump restaurant logo to take home with them as a special memory.

While Francis was at his last Fourth of July church picnic (Hamilton's annual picnic at Boothbay Park, south of San Francisco), he received a call from Betty and Ruth who had left for home a couple of days earlier. They had stopped off at the Best Friends animal rescue sanctuary somewhere in Utah, where they adopted a chocolate lab named Cocoa-Latte. All the Smiths were animal nuts, and Cocoa would surely fit right in! With their new happy canine companion in tow, they finished their last leg home to Fort Wayne, Indiana.

Later that July, Francis attended what would be his last lab picnic in South San Francisco, overlooking San Francisco International Airport. He brought along his favorite tried and true recipe of homemade macaroni and cheese, which was an immediate hit. For him, it was a bittersweet time of success and farewells.

Now it was time to schedule his oral defense of his dissertation in the form of a seminar open to the faculty and students at UCSF along with anyone else that was interested in one of the main lecture theaters. He was able to schedule it for midmorning of August 28.

Those last few weeks in August were busy ones. Francis attended his last church service where he said goodbye to his church family as well as to other dear friendships he had developed over the years in the City by the Bay. Saying goodbye is always difficult, so instead, it was "See you later."

> *Beloved, let us love one another, for love is from God, and whoever loves has been born of God and knows God.*
> —1 John 4:7

Chapter 3

The Everlasting Way

Search me, O God, and know my heart:
Try me and know my anxious thoughts;
And see if there be any hurtful way in me,
And lead me in the everlasting way.

—Psalm 139:23–24

Francis Finishes the Race
San Francisco, California (August 28, 2012)

Francis was slumbering when he felt a tap on his shoulder. He awoke with a start. Sitting on his briefcase with his arms folded across his chest was King Brian.

"Get up you lazy bum," King Brian said with his thick Irish brogue. "Ye are almost there!"

Francis rubbed the sleep out of his eyes and looked around. Had he heard something? On his Bible, he noticed, was a note. Curious, he picked it up. In large, Celtic-style letters it said, "Congratulations! Ye followed the narrow road. Ye found the Pot o' Gold." It was signed, "Ye Old Friend Forever, King Brian."

Francis chuckled. Yes, he thought to himself, he certainly had followed the narrow road and *his* Pot o' Gold was the LORD's free gift of eternal life. Gently he folded the note and placed it inside his Bible. What a wonderful day! In those quiet moments, the LORD had indeed searched his heart. He even knew his anxious thoughts, and His presence was calming. Shaking off his nerves, he gathered his belongings and headed out the door. The short walk from his apartment to the UCSF campus afforded him time to enjoy the beauty of the warm summer day while losing himself in thoughts of God's grace and mercy that carried him through so many seemingly insurmountable odds to lead him to this special day. Through hindsight, there was no doubt in his mind that the LORD's hand had been on his life from the moment he was conceived.

The unwitting nudges and stares that followed Francis wherever he went no longer affected him, for he had come to terms with his physical differences a very long time ago. The years of bullying he had endured only served to strengthen him and cause him to lean on the LORD even more although the process was debilitating at the time. Francis knew that, in God's eyes, he was perfect because God had formed him for His purpose alone, not for that of the world's. (After all, when it comes to this world, Francis was just passing through!) The LORD had seen to it that he was given a family that not only taught him to love the LORD but to make Him his priority in all things. The LORD did, indeed, have plans for Francis. All he had to do was listen carefully, walk in obedience, and trust in His wisdom; and from there, the LORD would work out the rest. What God gave him in great abundance was a heart to encourage others that suffered, as he had, with craniofacial anomalies.

There were a goodly number of audience members already inside the lecture theatre when Francis arrived. He tried with great difficulty to squelch the butterflies that threatened to fly out of his stomach. After all, this was the dream he had strived toward for the last twenty out of his thirty-seven years. After personally greeting as many guests he could, he delivered his seminar in front of faculty members, peers, students, committee members, and a few close friends, Don and Karen Maalona and Michele DuBroy (who is the coauthor of this book), from church who came to listen and to support him. Concluding his talk and defense of his dissertation in response to questions from the audience, he had successfully delivered his dissertation. After, he enjoyed a huge sense of relief and gave thanks for the LORD who carried him through his talk. All that was left to do was to make some minor revisions and submit it again.

Meanwhile, back in Fort Wayne, Indiana, Betty and Ruth prayed diligently for Francis's special day. Betty was so excited she could barely eat a thing, and waiting to hear from Francis had made each minute seem like hours. When the call finally came, they were both over the moon. "I've always felt very blessed with my children. I was so excited. We were elated." Ruth has also had tremendous successes.

"I am the most blessed mother on the planet with the kids I've got. The LORD answered my prayers for a family, guidance, and protection; and He provided the way and orchestrated the plan, and he gave us all many miracles," mentioned Betty in complete humility.

***

Francis's last week in San Francisco was busy with packing up his clothes and housewares and putting whatever he couldn't pack into his car in storage and getting his car checked out for the epic long road trip northbound toward Calgary.

Moving day arrived at the very end of August. That evening after he finished cleaning his flat and handing over the apartment keys to the housing office, Francis began the grand five-day road trip to Calgary. Through California, Oregon, and Washington, he steadily trekked before heading eastward into Idaho, where he eventually turned northward where he crossed the Canadian border into British Colombia and eastward again into Alberta, arriving in Calgary on the American holiday, Labor Day.

That fall while in Calgary, Francis received the official word from UCSF that he had received his doctorate, a PhD in craniofacial research, and later on, he received his diploma via mail. With his doctorate in hand, he heads into a new era of praise and thanks, service, and adventure, continuing to go boldly wherever the LORD leads.

***

Dr. Francis Joel Smith

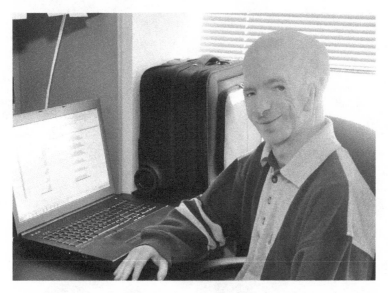

Dr. Smith, University of Colorado

Beam me up, Jesus!

I have fought a good fight,
I have finished the race,
I have kept the faith.

—2 Timothy 4:7

Let your light shine before men in such a way that they may see
your good works, and glorify your Father who is in heaven.

—Matthew 5:6

Reflection

From the time Francis was brought into the God-fearing, God-loving Smith family where he was taught to love the LORD with all his heart, he was also encouraged to never give into his challenges. No matter what, the LORD was revered for His perfect plan He had orchestrated for Francis from the moment he was conceived. Francis's challenges were for God's purpose and glory, as He is "in everything." Over time, in spite of missteps, numerous setbacks that were sometimes the result of his own willfulness, Francis was able to embrace God's magnificent grace in all his difficulties. What enabled him to do this was his own unwavering faith, prayer and fellowship, and praise in all things. Francis's ongoing prayer for others who are challenged is that they will soon embrace God's perfect plan for their own lives. God designed each of us in our mother's womb exactly as He planned. He planned the color of our eyes, the color of our skin—everything about us. After all, God does not make mistakes!

Father, forgive me for not agreeing with You that I am fearfully and wonderfully made. Forgive me for believing the lies that I have to be somebody other than who I am. Help me to come into agreement with Your love for me and not despise all my imperfections. The fact that You love me and accept me is more important than the love and acceptance from anyone else. I am thankful that I am Your child, and that I am fearfully and wonderfully made! I know that full well. In the name of Your beloved Son Jesus I pray. Amen.

—Unknown

Afterword from the Professors

Dr. Ralph Marcucio

I met Francis in 2007 when he came to speak with me about applying to graduate school at the University of California San Francisco. This is not an uncommon event. My area of expertise is the study craniofacial birth defects. Although I was aware that Francis had Treacher Collins syndrome (TCS), I had never actually met anyone who is afflicted with it, and I was concerned about how I was going to react. Little did I know at that time how knowing Francis was going to change both my professional and personal life.

Upon meeting Francis, my qualms quickly faded as his enthusiasm and passion drove the conversation. There was no doubt in my mind during that meeting that Francis belonged in our craniofacial research program, and immediately, I became his PhD advisor and scientific mentor. Francis did not waste any time taking the bull by the horns. One of the first things he accomplished was to design and build a special incubator he needed for his experiments on oxygen and birth defects, and from there, he painstakingly, one day at a time, one step at a time, began to travel the long difficult road toward completing his PhD dissertation research. I was humbled by his dedication and work ethic that never once wavered.

While working with Francis every weekday for the next five years, our work relationship developed into a friendship. In short order, he proved to be an exciting addition to my laboratory, and he was a pleasure to advise. Everybody loved him. He is funny, gracious, polite, and stubborn. He eats enormous amounts of food, collects skulls, has a fondness of extraterrestrials, and plays a green violin; and he's not shy about reaching out to anyone who crosses his path, personally and professionally. As his mentor responsible for his training, I was more than pleased because Francis was an exemplary, hardworking student who was completely driven to complete his PhD.

Watching Francis develop from a first-year graduate student into a member of the craniofacial research community was a very rewarding process. Toward the end of his time in my laboratory, we attended a meeting on craniofacial biology. While several of us sat around a table talking about science and having fun in a local pub, Francis sat down at the piano and entertained everyone with his vast musical repertoire. A fun evening was turned into a memorable evening that is still talked about by all of us who were there. Francis's friendly, outgoing, and humorous personality, not to mention his intellect, captivates just about everyone. No one remembers when he became fully integrated into our scientific community because there was never a time when he wasn't, or so it seems.

Francis taught me what we have all been told: look beyond appearance, appreciate diversity, and consider our fortunes good. Francis is my inspiration as I hope he will be yours. My hope is that his story inspires others to tackle challenges like Francis does, to set the bar high the way Francis does, and to embrace life like Francis does.

Dr. John Greenspan

At the time I met Francis, I was the associate dean for Research and Graduate Affairs at the UCSF, and I was asked to meet him, mostly because of our King's College London connection. I was aware then that several faculty members were reluctant to take him on. I too was concerned.

Upon meeting Francis, I took an immediate liking to him. He displayed an amazing motivation and was obviously quite undeterred by his situation, about which he spoke cheerfully and objectively. Whatever concerns I had about him were immediately put behind me and never addressed again. From that moment on, I did what I could to support his entry here, and he worked with Daniel Ramos, who also sort of adopted him.

Francis, in very short order, rose to the occasion and endeared himself to all he encountered. We have watched his progress with admiration and pride, for he continues to overcome his TCS and to excel, carving a very special niche in academic craniofacial science and community outreach. I am proud to know and be associated with Francis.

Dr. Daniel Ramos

I was asked by Dr. John Greenspan to attend a seminar given by Francis in 2007. The speaker was Francis Smith who was presenting his MS work he had just completed at King's College in London. At the time, I was on the steering committee for the graduate program in orofacial sciences. I met with him and thought he would be a wonderful addition to the program. I was so impressed with Francis that I hosted his first rotation at UCSF. I immediately was drawn to his beautiful spirit. My group taught Francis how to perform immunofluorescence microscopy, and he excelled. This was no mere feat as the person teaching Francis did not speak English very well, and with his hearing problems, it could have become a problem. Instead, for the first few weeks, we would just e-mail our technical conversations, and *problem solved.*

He became friends with my two teenage sons. We had him over for a July 4 holiday, just weeks after he arrived, and he immediately started to develop a sense of community. One of the things that Francis, my girlfriend Nancy, and I bonded over was baseball. We went to many San Francisco Giants games, and still when he visits San Francisco, we try to catch a game. I had the pleasure of meeting his mother who is also an incredible person. Francis has become such a force in craniofacial biology, but to me, he will always be Franny. It has been quite an honor as well as a lot of fun to know Francis.

A Note from the Author, Michele DuBroy

When I first met Francis in 2008 when we were both attending Hamilton Square Baptist Church in San Francisco and where I still attend today, I couldn't help but be completely mesmerized by this outwardly different-looking but somehow completely captivating young man whose outward joy was apparently quite contagious. Although it took some time for us to settle into a friendship, it was difficult not to notice the wonderful ongoing effect Francis has on people. What was his appeal? I often pondered.

Francis's appeal, I soon discovered, is his joy and outright reverence for the LORD that shines ever so brightly from within him. Like a moth is drawn to the flame, people are drawn to him.

After finally completing this years-long journey of researching and crafting his story, I am thoroughly convinced that Francis's relationship with his personal LORD and Savior, Jesus, began way back in his mother's womb where he was being knitted to perfection for the LORD's divine purpose during his earthly life. God foreknew all along exactly the plans He had for Francis.

Being an author/writer with numerous publishing credits, naturally I soon came to realize that Francis was a walking, talking, breathing testimony waiting to be told. During the course of our friendship, little bits and pieces kept surfacing when finally the seed that was planted had grown so large inside me it was impossible to ignore. After learning that Francis had written numerous and meticulous pages about his life journey, we finally discussed the possibility of turning his life story into a book.

A huge part of an author/writer's job is research, and I have passed through this phase countless times—but this time was different. This time, a great deal of my research took place in God's Word, and no one can spend time in God's Word without embarking on an incredible transformational journey. The LORD had my rapt attention, and He used that time to complete a great deal of His miraculous fine-tuning in my own life. Believe me, I needed it!

One amazing perk of writing this story were the countless hours I got to spend talking primarily with Betty and also with Ruth and the two memorable summertime visits to their home in Fort Wayne, Indiana. By then, Betty was in her early nineties, and along with Ruth, the two of them were caring for James's young grandson who himself suffered from the same birth challenges that James did. Even at her advanced age, Betty was doing what she did best, caring for challenged children others would have given up on. After getting to know Betty well enough to consider her to be my own "adopted" mother, I was not surprised to see her give her great-grandson the same love and guidance she had given her now-adult children during her earlier years. Ruth was just as involved with her nephew even though she was still completing school for her degree and working a full-time job. They were a dedicated team.

My curiosity-driven questions were probing. I cannot imagine how difficult it was for Betty to so willingly revisit the past, which at times was excruciatingly painful. Never one to shy away from the pain that life often deals out, she readily admits that no matter how sorrowful certain phases of her life were, the LORD never once failed to turn those sad times around and turn it into something good. Much of her pain was used to strengthen and refine and prepare her for the innumerable blessings and miracles He planned for her. There were many tears during our journey, but all throughout the ups and downs, her trust in the LORD remained unshakable, a trait she did her best to pass on to her family

This proved to be a far more difficult journey that I was prepared for. There is nothing Satan hates more than when someone sets out to do the LORD's work, especially when that work is going to affect multitudes of people. On two different occasions, my setbacks were so devastating I felt I couldn't possibly be the one to tell this remarkable story. After the second setback, I ended up in Pastor Innes's office, near tears, explaining why I couldn't possibly continue on with my work. Expecting tea and sympathy along with some pastorly understanding, what I got instead was his very wise and biblical counsel. "Pick yourself back up, brush yourself off, and start all over again," he said. *What?* Who am I to argue with my pastor? With great reluctance and riding on my own and the many prayers of others for guidance, I did exactly that. As my friends Christa and Steve from my Bible study group pointed out, this newer version is far superior to the work I had previously done. Once again, the devil was thwarted. And now, in God's perfect timing and for His specific divine purpose, this body of work has finally come to fruition.

My prayer for everyone who reads Francis's amazing story is that each and every one of you will be encouraged to examine your own heart, and if you don't already know the LORD personally, you will answer His knock. It's never too late, and there is no sin too big for Him not to forgive. He is standing at your door. We are all sinners who are in desperate need of a Savior. Acknowledge your sins, confess them, and invite Jesus into your life. Jesus will do the rest. The outcome of your decision will be eternal.

The Smith Family

Andrew, Betty's only biological child, was born in 1947. After serving in Vietnam, he returned home with a severe case of posttraumatic stress disorder. Shortly after his return, he disappeared. After years of fruitless searching for him, it was finally discovered that he passed away in 1996 in Sacramento, California, after being hit by a car while walking across a road.

Billy, Bob and Betty's first adopted child, in 1961, at four years old, was officially "unadopted" due to a deteriorating psychotic mental illness.

Edwin, adopted in 1962, is happily married and a father.

Peter, adopted in 1962, died two days after a head-on collision in September 1982. He was newly engaged to be married.

Angel, adopted in 1962, passed away from cancer in 2016. Angel is survived by her beloved husband and their three adult children.

Susie, adopted in 1963, is married and the parent of three adult children.

Rob and Rebecca, twins, were adopted in 1966. Rob was divorced with two children but is now happily married to his second wife, Linda. Rebecca is also married with children.

James, adopted in 1969, was incarcerated for drug dealing. While there, he restored his faith in God and as a result became the assistant to the prison chaplain. In 2017, James was released from prison and now successfully manages a halfway house for other former addicts who are moving forward with their lives.

Christopher, adopted in 1970, is now happily married with children.

Ruth Smith, adopted in 1983 at three years old, has achieved her master's degree in psychology and went on to become Ms. Wheelchair Indiana for two years, 2014–2015, and is a job placement counselor for people with special needs.

Betty Smith, in her nineties, still lives independently in her Fort Wayne home, and Ruth lives at home with her to help her out. Both are caring for James's young grandson, Jaxzin.

Current Events in Francis's Life

Francis remains very close to his mother and his sister Ruth, and once (or more) a year, he travels home to visit her in Fort Wayne, usually at Christmas, but sometimes also for family reasons (such as Angel's funeral in 2016, Rob's second wedding later that year, and, once in a while, just to sneak up on and surprise Betty).

Since completing his PhD, Francis remains busy with his craniofacial research and public engagements activities to raise awareness of craniofacial anomalies and foster acceptance of those affected by these conditions.

Currently, Francis is in his second postdoctoral fellowship at the University of Colorado medical campus in Aurora (a suburb of Denver). This fellowship will end in 2018, so he is currently searching for his next position somewhere on earth where he plans to combine research with public outreach. He is also working on writing his own NIH grant so he can stay on a few more years in Denver, if successfully funded.

Public outreach to raise awareness of craniofacial conditions and the need for continuing research remains a personal passion that is dear to Francis's heart. He continues to be interviewed on radio and television and often speaks at various venues, including schools, churches, and meetings. CCA and Cher's Family Retreat, however, remain a regular event in his life. On the CCA website, he has his own regular feature blog, known as *From the Bench with Francis*, where he updates the CCA audience with news from the craniofacial scientific and medical world along with his own reflections. He is also a member of a group that organizes and hosts a biannual "Fabulous Faces at Sea Craniofacial Cruises" event where those with craniofacial anomalies can get away on a cruise that includes group-specific shipboard activities and shore excursions.

Travel, to this day, remains a significant part of Francis's life. Regularly, he accepts any invitations that are possible for him to speak or to videotape interviews of his former research partners or simply to attend international craniofacial conferences. For the latter half of 2017, his plans are to visit three different countries—Australia; back to England and King's College and a university in Norwich, England; and a major craniofacial research hospital in Bauru, Brazil.

In early 2017, he traveled back to Indianapolis to revisit one of his hospital alma maters, Riley Hospital for Children, as well as Camp About Face. In Cincinnati, Ohio, in late June, he attended a Treacher Collins syndrome symposium; then he was off to the next CCA retreat in Washington DC.

Music remains of utmost importance in his life, and he regularly plays the piano, green violin, and guitar. Photography also remains an important hobby that he enjoys, not to mention his love of antiquing (medical and otherwise).

On the spiritual front, Francis remains faithful and active in churches. Currently in Denver, he attends Beth Eden Baptist Church that he found with help from Pastor

Innes at Hamilton Square Baptist Church in San Francisco, who is friends with its pastor, Jason Pilchard. There, he remains active in his music ministry. Francis hangs on tenaciously to his strong faith in Christ, trusting him to guide him to the next steps in his earthly journey. He also hangs on each and every day to the promises in God's Word.

Last but not least, during his most recent trip back to the Indianapolis area, he took it upon himself to visit his old childhood haunts. He had taken some time to research Mrs. Collins's death and burial. She passed away on August 26, 1992, from emphysema and was buried in a southwest Indianapolis cemetery, Floral Park Cemetery, on August 29 of that same year. Francis visited her grave where he was finally able to achieve closure with a visit to his dear foster mother's grave. While there, he thanked the LORD for orchestrating their time together, a time that provided a great stepping stone to starting a lifetime of God's love and purpose.

Francis's lifelong prayer of meeting his biological birth parents and their family has yet to be achieved. But he remains prayerful that the LORD, in His perfect timing, will open that door. He will never think of anyone else than Betty and Bob as his God-given parents, but God also chose his birth parents to bring him into the world, and he would like to thank them.

Amazing Grace
John Newton

Amazing grace
How sweet the sound
That saved a wretch like me
I once was lost, but now I'm found
'Twas grace that taught my heart to fear
And grace my fears relieved
How precious did that grace appear
The hour I first believed
My chains are gone
I've been set free
My God, my Savior has ransomed me
And like a flood His mercy rains
Unending love, Amazing grace.

The Smith Children
Order of Adoption

1947—Andrew is born, the first and only biological child of Betty and her first husband who passed away. Adopted by Bob Smith.

1961—Billy, four years old

1962—Edwin, eight years old

1962—Peter, one year old, Hopi Indian

1962—Angel, five days old, South American

1963—Susie, seven months old

1966—Rob and Rebecca, five months old

1969—James, newborn, biracial

1970—Christopher, ten months, biracial

1977—Hugh Dermot O'Connor or Francis Joel Smith, two and a half years old

1984—Ruth or Delana, three years old

Francis Smith's Medical History

List of Surgeries/Hospitalizations

1975

April 25: Birth at Bloomington Hospital, Bloomington, Indiana; transferred to James Whitcomb Riley Hospital for Children in Indianapolis.

April 25–June 6: First, emergency tracheotomy at age one day (April 26) after respiratory arrest and inability to insert a breathing tube by mouth (tracheotomy kept in place for next five years); multiple resuscitations for respiratory arrest due to blocked airway. Long stint in neonatal intensive care unit at Riley Hospital.

Turned over to Mrs. Collins for foster care in Indianapolis.

November 24–December 6: Hospitalized at Riley Hospital for failure to thrive (malnutrition, recurrent vomiting, inability to feed, severe underweight).

1978

May 9: Palate repair by Dr. Singer.

Anesthesia: General, through tracheotomy.

Hospitalized for little over a week (Riley Hospital).

August 2: Two-part surgery: 1) Partial closure of oral-nasal fistula (hole) remaining from previous palate repair. 2) Exploration of left middle ear, unable to open atresia (total blockage by bone) of ear canal; there were no usable middle ear structures, so it was decided unfeasible to reconstruct ear canals without damaging what little I had left of ears. Done by Dr. Tubergen.

Anesthesia: General, through tracheotomy.

Hospitalized for a week (Riley Hospital).

1978 or 1979

Date unknown: Dental procedure (under nitrous oxide gas anesthesia?) at pediatric dentist's office in Fort Wayne, Indiana; nearly died from respiratory arrest in the chair and had to be resuscitated by EMTs and firefighters. From then on, all dental care was undertaken at Riley Hospital dental clinic.

1979

December 9: Decannulation (removal of tracheotomy tube, but hole remained open. Hospitalized for four days (Riley Hospital).

1980

August 14: Failed attempt to close tracheal opening, after multiple attempts to intubate (insert a breathing tube) orally during general anesthesia for procedure. Tracheotomy tube placed temporarily. Three-day stay (Riley Hospital).

1982

May: Craniofacial surgical care transferred to Dr. Jeffrey Marsh and his multidisciplinary team (Cleft Palate and Craniofacial Deformities Institute) at St. Louis Children's Hospital, St. Louis, Missouri; preliminary evaluations by entire team; set up surgical plan.

July and August: Long hospitalization (four weeks) at St. Louis Children's Hospital, with two surgeries back-to-back (separated by a week or two).

First surgery—attempt to repair fistula (hole left over from palate repair in 1978) in palate with tongue flap (part of tongue with one end over hole in palate, other end still attached to tongue). Tongue flap came loose from palate within a week of surgery, necessitating emergency blood transfusion. Lived with lump on surface of tongue for the next five years until next attempt.

Anesthesia: General, through mask.

Second surgery—lower jaw split on each side and realigned. Jaws wired shut for two months. Tracheostomy (left in place for two months). Two days in oxygen tent in ICU.

Anesthesia: General, through mask, then tracheostomy.

Both surgeries were done by Dr. Marsh's team.

Went home late August for about a month.

September: Returned to St. Louis for removal of wires holding jaws shut and removal of tracheotomy, under general anesthesia. Done by Dr. Marsh's team.

"Legend of the Pancake Kid" poem takes place at this time, which tells story of how I wanted pancakes for my first solid meal after having my jaw wires removed (I had been eating everything as blenderized liquid food through a large syringe while my jaws were wired shut).

1983

May: Reconstruction of missing cheekbones and lower eye socket rims with rib grafts and wires and screws;

possibly when my right eye went nearly totally blind for life. Also, first earlobe reconstruction. Dr. Marsh and team (St. Louis Children's Hospital).

Anesthesia: General, through mask.

October: Second stage of ear reconstruction: rib and pelvic skin grafts used to create first-stage earlobes. Dr. Marsh and team (St. Louis Children's Hospital).

Anesthesia: General, through mask.

1984

May 9: Dental procedure under general anesthesia to put crowns on three teeth, along with dental impressions for a planned future palate speech appliance. Very difficult nasal-tracheal intubation for anesthesia (I still remember waking up repeatedly during the procedure). Due to very difficult anesthesia, I had to stay one night after the procedure (Riley Hospital).

Fall: Third-stage earlobe reconstruction. Dr. Marsh and team (St. Louis Children's Hospital).

Anesthesia: General, through mask.

1985

July: Comprehensive outpatient evaluation by entire team at St. Louis Children's Hospital, planning for next few years of surgeries.

1986

January: Surgical procedure for ear reconstruction aborted due to unsuccessful attempt to insert endotracheal tube by mouth into my throat during induction of general anesthesia after I had been put to sleep with the Mask (my throat is too narrow to allow anesthesiologists to see my vocal cords in order to insert a tube to breathe for me during surgery). Dr. Marsh and team (St. Louis Children's Hospital).

May (Mother's Day): Choked nearly to death on sausage during breakfast at Auburn, Indiana, Ponderosa buffet steak house restaurant; transferred from Auburn's DeKalb Memorial Hospital to Riley Hospital in Indianapolis by ambulance.

July: Major lower jaw reconstruction involving splitting jaw on each side and repositioning using special-shaped metal plates and screws. Tracheotomy inserted during procedure (left in place for six weeks) and jaws wired tightly shut for six weeks. Hospitalized for over a week, sent home for six weeks with trache and wired-shut jaws and syringe-fed liquid diet. Dr. Marsh and team (St. Louis Children's Hospital).

Anesthesia: General, through mask, then tracheotomy.

During that six-week recovery period at home, tracheotomy tube came out of my throat one night, and I was rushed to Fort Wayne, Indiana, Parkview Memorial Hospital Emergency Room, and it could not be put back in (hole started to close up already); I somehow managed to breathe from then on without it.

September: Removal of jaw fixation wires under general anesthesia. Dr. Marsh and team (St. Louis Children's Hospital).

1987

March 3: Implantation of magnetic plate for Xomed Audiant implantable bone conduction hearing aid behind left ear. First "same-day" surgery for me (done on day of admission; previous ones had been done day after admission). Done by Dr. Miyamoto, ear, nose, and throat surgeon. Hospitalized overnight after procedure (Riley Hospital).

Anesthesia: General, through IV, then intubation.

March: Comprehensive all-team evaluation at St. Louis Children's Hospital.

June: Upper jaw reconstruction and second attempt at tongue flap repair of palatal fistula (this time, it stayed up there), lump of tongue sewn to palate while still attached to tongue (would stay together that way for six weeks), and tracheotomy. Dr. Marsh and team (St. Louis Children's Hospital).

Anesthesia: General, through mask, then tracheotomy.

August: Removal of tongue from palate, leaving tongue flap in place on palate, and removal of tracheotomy, under general anesthesia. Dr. Marsh and team (St. Louis Children's Hospital).

1988

Spring: Comprehensive all-team evaluation at St. Louis Children's Hospital.

July: Final stage of earlobe reconstruction. Dr. Marsh and team (St. Louis Children's Hospital).

Anesthesia: General, through mask.

1989, 1990, 1991

Multiple visits to St. Louis Children's Hospital for team evaluation (no actual surgeries during this time). Decision to return my craniofacial care to Riley Hospital in Indianapolis from then on.

1991

December 4: Marathon fourteen-hour lower jaw reconstruction procedure involving rib grafts with cartilage on the end of each to provide a ball joint on each side as well as repositioning jaw. Jaws wired shut tightly with wires. Tracheotomy inserted, after I was put to sleep with the Mask (the last time the Mask was used on me). Jaws wired shut for two months solid; tracheotomy kept in place for about two weeks. First night in ICU, nearly asphyxiated to death when tracheotomy completely plugged up (and no response to repeated frantic attempts to call nurses with call button while all alone in ICU cubicle). Done by Dr. Nelson and Dr. Hayhurst, both maxillofacial surgeons (Riley Hospital).

Anesthesia: General, through mask (the last time mask was used on me), then tracheotomy.

Jaw wires removed in February 1992 under sedation in oral surgery office at Long Hospital (near Riley Hospital) in Indianapolis.

1992

July: Upper jaw reconstruction. Drs. Nelson and Hayhurst (Riley Hospital).

Anesthesia: General, via awake fiberoptic intubation. (This was the first time I was kept awake while anesthesiologists inserted breathing tube in my throat using fiberoptic scope to guide them, called fiberoptic awake intubation; used as standard anesthetic induction procedure on me from then on.)

1993

March 26: Two-part surgery: 1) Insertion of custom-made shaped white porous facial contour implants in chin and under both eyes (Dr. Eppley and plastic surgery team). 2) Eye muscle shortening surgery for right eye (Dr. Helveston, ophthalmic surgeon). Hospitalized overnight after surgery (Riley Hospital).

Anesthesia: General, via IV, then intubation with a special airway called LMA (laryngeal mask airway, a short "pig-snout" airway that can be blindly inserted).

April 20: Emergency surgery to drain and clean out infection in right eye implant; whole week in hospital (April 19–26) under strong IV antibiotic therapy. Eighteenth birthday spent in hospital. Dr. Eppley (Riley Hospital).

1994

July 14: Biopsy of right side of jaw for suspicious opaque area seen in dental X-ray; done with local anesthesia in oral surgery at Indiana University Hospital, Indianapolis.

Found it was not cancer (as suspected to be) but old scar tissue in bone from multiple previous jaw surgeries.

1995

June 29: Second emergency surgery for recurrent infection of one of my facial contour implants, this time on left side; drained and irrigated under general anesthesia. Weeklong hospitalization for strong IV antibiotic therapy. Dr. Eppley (Riley Hospital).

Anesthesia: General, via awake fiberoptic intubation.

December 31: Another emergency early-in-the-morning surgery for recurrent left-implant infection on New Year's Eve at Riley Hospital (with a skeleton crew there); released same day. Dr. Eppley.

Anesthesia: General, via awake fiberoptic intubation.

1996

March 4: Yet another emergency surgery to drain and irrigate a recurring infection in left implant under eye; weeklong hospitalization under strong IV antibiotic therapy. Dr. Eppley (Riley Hospital).

Anesthesia: General, via awake fiberoptic intubation.

August 12: Left implant finally removed and site drained and irrigated (to prevent further recurrence of infection). Dr. Eppley. Released same day (Riley Hospital).

Anesthesia: General, via awake fiberoptic intubation.

2003

September 26: Implantation of screw behind right ear for BAHA (bone-anchored hearing aid) implantable hearing device under general anesthesia. Dr. Tubergen. Released same day (St. Vincent Hospital, Indianapolis).

Anesthesia: General, via IV, then intubation with LMA.

About the Author

Michele DuBroy has been published in over four hundred news publications, magazines, e-zines, and trade publications as a writer, photographer, staff, and feature writer. She often publishes pseudonymously, and her book—*Donkey Galloping Out of Hell (as M. M. Harris)*, the true story of Luftwaffe pilot Jack Hildebrandt—is critically acclaimed and has been excerpted in several World War II high-gloss publications.

Michele met Francis when they both attended Hamilton Square Baptist Church in San Francisco where she became a member in 2006. Since 2007, Michele has worked as a para professional II in the special education department at a Bay Area high school and is a strong advocate for those with special needs. After losing her own mother, Margaret, in 2009, she considers Betty Smith to be her own adopted mother. How fitting that Margaret and Betty share the same birthday, September 23.

Michele is currently working on the screenplay version of this book.

About the Photographer

Faculty Trustee
Kenneth Bisio was elected to the MSU Denver Board
of Trustees in 2014 and re-elected in 2015 and 2016.

Kenn is a full professor of Journalism and Technical
Communication at Metropolitan State University of
Denver where he teaches Photojournalism and Social
Documentary. He is also a world-renowned photojournalist with more than 40 years as a working pro. His images
have been published worldwide in popular and prestigious
newspapers and magazines for which he has received
numerous awards. His photographs have been displayed
in exhibits in America, Europe, Russia, and the Far East
and are purchased by individual, corporate, museum, and
gallery collectors. Kenn's photographs are also in the NFL
Hall of Fame for his coverage of four Super Bowls. He
is represented by the Geraint Smith Gallery in Taos, New
Mexico.

CPSIA information can be obtained
at www.ICGtesting.com
Printed in the USA
JSHW022305180822
29398JS00006B/2